Pioneering Human Myoblast Genome Therapy

PIONEERING HUMAN MYOBLAST GENOME THERAPY

PETER K. LAW, DANLIN M. LAW
PING LU, EUGENE K. W. SIM,
KHAWJA H. HAIDER, LEI YE,
XUN LI, MARGARITA N. VAKHROMEEVA,
ILIA I. BERISHVILLI
AND
LEO A. BOCKERIA

Nova Biomedical Books
New York

For permission to use material from this book please contact us:
Telephone 631-231-7269; Fax 631-231-8175
Web Site: http://www.novapublishers.com

NOTICE TO THE READER

The Publisher has taken reasonable care in the preparation of this book, but makes no expressed or implied warranty of any kind and assumes no responsibility for any errors or omissions. No liability is assumed for incidental or consequential damages in connection with or arising out of information contained in this book. The Publisher shall not be liable for any special, consequential, or exemplary damages resulting, in whole or in part, from the readers' use of, or reliance upon, this material.

Independent verification should be sought for any data, advice or recommendations contained in this book. In addition, no responsibility is assumed by the publisher for any injury and/or damage to persons or property arising from any methods, products, instructions, ideas or otherwise contained in this publication.

This publication is designed to provide accurate and authoritative information with regard to the subject matter covered herein. It is sold with the clear understanding that the Publisher is not engaged in rendering legal or any other professional services. If legal or any other expert assistance is required, the services of a competent person should be sought. FROM A DECLARATION OF PARTICIPANTS JOINTLY ADOPTED BY A COMMITTEE OF THE AMERICAN BAR ASSOCIATION AND A COMMITTEE OF PUBLISHERS.

LIBRARY OF CONGRESS CATALOGING-IN-PUBLICATION DATA

ISBN: 978-1-60692-817-2

Available upon request

Published by Nova Science Publishers, Inc. ✛ *New York*

CONTENTS

PREFACE

Human Myoblast Genome Therapy (HMGT) is a platform technology of cell transplantation, nuclear transfer, and tissue engineering. Myoblasts are differentiated, immature cells destined to become muscles. Myoblasts cultured from muscle biopsy survive, develop and function to revitalize degenerative muscles upon transplantation. Transplant injury activates regeneration of host myofibers that fuse with the injected myoblasts, sharing their nuclei in a common gene pool of the syncytium. Thus, through nuclear transfer and complementation, human genome can be transferred into muscles of genetically-ill patients to achieve phenotype repair. Myoblasts are safe and efficient universal gene transfer vehicles endogenous to muscles that constitute 50% of the body. Myoblasts fuse among themselves to form new myofibers. Patients take only 2-month cyclosporine to immunosuppress allograft rejection because myofibers do not express MHC-1 antigens.

The first correction of human gene defect was published in the Lancet on July 14, 1990 when the therapeutic protein dystrophin was found in the myoblast-injected muscle of a Duchenne muscular dystrophy (DMD) patient. Results over 280 HMGT procedures on MD subjects in the past 15 years demonstrated absolute safety. Myoblast-injected DMD muscles showed improved histology. Strength increase at 18 months post-operatively averaged 123%. FDA-approved clinical trials progressed unto Phase III in USA with direct cost recovery.

Heart muscle degeneration is the leading cause of human debilitation and death. The first human myoblast transfer into porcine myocardium in May 2000 revealed that it was safe to administer one billion myoblasts at 10^8/ml using 20 injections inside the left ventricle. Surgical HMGT into 50 infarcted porcine hearts demonstrated three mechanisms as proof of concept. Some myoblasts trans-differentiated to become cardiomyocytes. Others transferred their nuclei into host cardiomyocytes through cell fusion. As yet others formed skeletal myofibers with satellite cells. *De novo* production of contractile filaments augmented heart contractility. Myoblasts transduced with VEGF165 and Angiopoeitin-1 genes produced six times more mature capillaries in infarcted porcine myocardium than placebo. Xenograft rejection was not observed for up to 30 weeks despite cyclosporine discontinuation at 6 weeks.

Clinical trials on approximately 150 severe heart patients in 12 countries demonstrated <10% mortality since June 2000. Most subjects received autologous cells implanted epicardially after CABG or endomyocardially. Two subjects each receiving 1-billion myoblast allograft and 2-month cyclosporine survived over one year. Significant increases in left ventricular ejection fraction, wall thickness and motion have been reported, with reduction in perfusion defective areas, angina and shortness of breath. Two European trials are in Phase II.

HMGT on two Type II diabetic subjects aimed to correct the GLUT4 genomic defects, producing insulin receptors on myofibers to facilitate glucose uptake for metabolism. Each subject received 24- billion allogenic myoblasts and 2-month cyclosporine. It has been 10 months and HMGT appears to be safe for both subjects.

Other HMGT targets include cosmetic enhancement, bone degeneration, cancer, anemia, hemophilia, human growth deficiency, muscle trauma, pain and depression. Transduced myoblasts and/or their derivatives act as stable bioreactor(s) to deliver long-term supplies of therapeutic protein(s) at optimal levels.

Chapter I

INTRODUCTION

This chapter is about the landmark development of a biomedical platform technology called Human Myoblast Genome Therapy (HMGT), known previously as Myoblast Transfer Therapy (MTT). The procedure of HMGT/MTT involves cell transplantation, nuclear transfer and tissue engineering to correct genetic defects and to strengthen degenerative and weak muscles.

Originally developed as a treatment for human muscular dystrophies in Phase III clinical trial in the USA, HMGT/MTT is now in Phase II clinical trials for treating heart failure in Europe, Phase I clinical trial for treating Type II diabetes in China, and tested for anti-aging cosmetic enhancement in Singapore.

This is the most up-to-date review by the pioneer of the technology, with critical evaluation of both basic experimentation and clinical trials. The conceptual approach and technological development are discussed. State-of-the-art methodology and results of the clinical trials are described in details with future perspectives. The work traverses the fields of genetics, neurology, pediatrics, cardiology, endocrinology, immunology, surgery, and developmental biology. HMGT/MTT will emerge as a mainstream platform technology of Regenerative Medicine.

DEVELOPMENT OF MAMMALIAN SKELETAL MUSCLES

Myoblasts

Mammalian skeletal muscles are derived from the mesodermal germ layer in the embryo. In human, mesoderm first appears at 20 days after fertilization [1]. Concomitant is the appearance of somites that increase in number with time. The somites provide the microenvironment in which the muscular system develops.

Within the somites are uncommitted mitotic stem cells capable of giving rise to muscle, bone, cartilage, blood, lymphatic, fat and connective tissues (Figure 1). The commitment to being myogenic occurs early on since myoblasts, as these cells are called, are found in the limb buds at 26 days of gestation. Satellite cells which are myoblast reserves in adult muscles contain actin-like filaments in their cytoplasm. Such lineage determination is influenced by embryonic induction and irreversible gene expression [2].

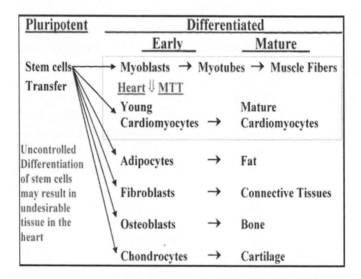

Figure 1. Pluripotent stem cells in the mesenchyme exhibit uncontrolled differentiation to become differentiated cells such as myoblasts, cardiomyocytes, fibroblasts, adipocytes, chondrocytes and osteoblasts. The benefits vs risk ratio of using myoblasts over stem cells in treating heart failure is greater. MTT, myoblast transfer therapy.

Lack of human fetal tissues for research in 1970s to 1980s has deemed myogenesis be studied in vitro. Figure 2 shows the different characteristics as the myoblasts develop. Beginning as small spheres of about 12 μm in diameter, myoblasts grow best on collagen attachment which somewhat resembles the extracellular matrix in vivo. Under proper culture condition, the transformation into spindle-shaped cells occurs within three days. These cells are characterized by their abilities to migrate, align, divide and fuse to form multinucleated myotubes that exhibit sarcomeres and immunostain positively for myosin. Equipped with these structural and biochemical bases of contraction, some myotubes can contract spontaneously in culture, and eventually pull from the culture surface. Without neural innervation the advance myotubes will undergo degeneration.

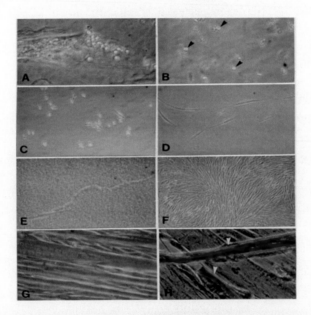

Figure 2. Human myogenic cell culture. (A) Satellite cells from human muscle biopsy. (B) Satellite cells 24 h after plating. (C) Satellite cells transforming to become spindle-shaped myoblasts at 48 h after plating. (D) Myoblasts at 96 h after plating. (E) Myoblast migrates. (F) Myoblasts align and confluent, ready for injection. (G) Higher magnification showing multi-nucleated myotubes with striations. (H) Myotubes immunostained with myosin antibody (arrowheads). One week after formation, spontaneously contracting myotubes detach from plate.

In the human fetus, close confinement within the somites ensures that the myoblasts are always at a state of confluence. The latter is a prerequisite for cell fusion. Cell division is an intrinsic property of myoblasts as evident by myoblast proliferation in serum-free culture media. However, proliferation in large quantity requires neurotrophic elements or factors [3,4]. It is known that myoblasts do not fuse when they are in the S, G2, M or even the early G1 phases of the cell cycle.

Although it is not possible to study division synchronization in the human fetus, it would appear to be a less important factor in myoblast fusion, considering that myoblast doubling time in culture is approximately 20 hours, and that myoblasts within a somite are essentially replicating clones.

Natural Cell Fusion

Reduction in serum or chick embryo extract concentration precipitates cell fusion in culture. Cell fusion occurs only after the myoblasts have undergone considerable cycles of division and are withdrawn from the mitotic cycle [3]. The decision to fuse in vivo is genetically programmed, and appears to occur without any neural contact or influence. It involves structural gene transcription and RNA synthesis, especially in the formation of the receptors on the myoblast surface that are responsible for cell recognition, cell adhesion, and membrane restructuring [4, 5]. The end product are multinucleated myotubes each of which is formed from fusion of 200 or more myoblasts.

Myotubes

Myotubes, with the many nuclei within the syncytium, are differentiated cells capable of producing large quantities of contractile proteins and related molecules. These proteins include, among others, myosin, actin, tropomyosin, and myoglobin. The contractile proteins are structured into filaments as the myotube develops, and are packaged into basic contracting units called the sarcomeres. Hundreds of sarcomeres are aligned to form a myofibril many of which comprise a myofiber. Each sarcomere is made up of myosin and actin filaments linked together by cross-bridges. Upon excitation-contraction coupling, millions of cross-bridges are formed, sliding the actin filaments toward the center of each myosin filament, and results in force generation [6]. Contraction and relaxation require $Ca2+$ and ATP, and membrane excitation needs innervation from motoneurons.

Myotube Maturation

The myotubes will not develop into a myofiber unless innervated by a motor axon. With the arrival of the axonal terminal, an area of the myotube membrane which is adjacent to the axonal terminal becomes thickened and convoluted due to the formation of large amounts of acetylcholine receptors and ionic channels. The mature neuromuscular junction is a highly specialized relay station, transmitting the central command to effect contraction of the myofiber. Neuromuscular transmission is through the release of the neuromuscular transmitter acetylcholine which, upon combining with their postjunctional receptors, is metabolized by cholinesterase and produces significant membrane depolarization to effect excitation-contraction [6]. These junctions stain positively for acetylcholinesterase.

As the bones elongate with age, the passive stretch induces additional sarcomere production with subsequent increase in strength. Although the number of myofibers remain constant for individual muscles, the number of myofibrils within the myofiber can vary according to genetic and environmental differences. As more contractile proteins are deposited and the sarcoplasmic reticulum better developed, the centrally located nuclei immigrate peripherally. Numerous structural proteins and glycoproteins are synthesized and deposited during the transition from myotube to myofiber. Among these is dystrophin, a surface membrane protein which is not present in the myofibers of Duchenne muscular dystrophy subjects [7] as a result of the genetic defect [8,9]. A built-in regenerative measure resides with the satellite cells that are basically myoblast reserves found in adult skeletal muscle fibers. These are mononucleated cells located between the basal lamina and the plasma membrane.

Broad Perspective

Like murine dystrophy, Duchenne muscular dystrophy (DMD) serves as a point of reference for us to test the Human Myoblast Genome Therapy (HMGT) as a treatment for hereditary muscle degenerative diseases. In a broad sense, HMGT is being developed to repair abnormal cells and to replenish dead cells of all degenerative and weak muscles. This has important implication in the development of treatments for muscle conditions exhibited in muscular dystrophies, heart muscle degeneration, Type II diabetes, aging and many others.

DUCHENNE MUSCULAR DYSTROPHY

The natural history of DMD depicts a continuous muscle degeneration and loss of strength, documented by subjective quantification [10-16], to begin at three years or younger, and continues throughout the course of the disease. Growth may outstrip the disease progress between four and five years of age, giving a false impression of remission or improvement; otherwise deterioration is continuous [11,17]. Degeneration is more severe in the proximal and anti-gravitational muscles than distal ones, and proximal muscle weakness in the lower body is responsible for the Gowers' sign used in physical diagnosis.

Debilitating and fatal, DMD affects 1 in 3300 live male births [18] and is the second most common lethal hereditary disease in human [19]. DMD individuals usually lose 50% of the strength in their leg muscles by age 9 due to muscle degeneration. They are wheelchair-bound by age 12, and three-quarters die before age 20. Pneumonia usually is the immediate cause of death, with underlying respiratory muscle degeneration, failure to inhale sufficient oxygen and to expel lung infection. Cardiomyopathic symptoms develop in mid adolescence [20] in about 10% of the DMD population. By age 18, all DMD individuals develop cardiomyopathy [21], but cardiac failure is seldom the primary cause of death [17].

The urgent need of a treatment for DMD prompted us to decide on using DMD in our initial clinical trials. We felt that if HMGT could benefit DMD individuals, it would likely benefit other muscle disease sufferers.

Murine Dystrophy Etiology-General Membrane Defect

The 129 ReJ-dydy [22] and the C57BL/6J dy2Jdy2J [23] dystrophic mice show autosomal recessive inheritance of dystrophy, with the dy mice having an earlier onset and a more rapid progression of the disease than the dy2J mice. Histopathology is similar to DMD, as is early death from respiratory failure due to muscle degeneration. Dystrophic symptoms appear at 3 to 4 weeks after birth and persist throughout the lives of these animals.

The *first* direct evidence of membrane abnormality in mammalian dystrophy was reported in 1972. The "cable" properties of normal and dy dystrophic mouse myofibers were compared using microelectrodes [24]. Subthreshold direct stimulation elicited a smaller response from the dystrophic fiber than from the normal one, indicating that the dystrophic fiber was "leaky" to the ionic current.

Subsequently, the ability of dystrophic muscle fibers to generate action potentials in response to supramaximal nerve stimulation was studied with intracellular microelectrodes. About 55% of the fibers examined were abnormal in their ability to generate action potentials. Some of these fibers showed no detectable response to stimulation of the motor nerve, whereas in others, abortive spikes or localized end-plate potentials were recorded. The proportion of fibers showing very small or no electrical response increased when recordings were made away from the end-plate zone. The abortive spikes indicated a structural defect in the sarcolemma such that sodium conductance was diminished [25].

The abortive spikes did not propagate the whole length of the myofibers such that sarcomeres further away from the motor end-plates would not receive depolarization to contract and would be wasted. Dystrophic myofibers with abortive spikes generated localized contraction close to the endplates but the tensions developed were lower than normal. Furthermore, when these fibers were subjected to the passive stretch of the antagonistic muscle and the active pull of the localized contraction, breach in the plasma membrane [26] might occur at the region of non-activated sarcomeres.

With leakage of Ca^{2+} into the myofibers, there are mitochrondrial Ca^{2+} overload and localized hypercontraction [28]. Also, Ca^{2+}-activated neutral proteases and lysosomal activities are activated resulting in muscle necrosis. Some fibers showed positive acid phospatase reaction in muscle nuclei, mitochondria, sarcoplasmic reticulum and contractile myofilaments [27]. Membrane defect was found not only in the sarcolemma, but also in the sarcoplasmic reticulum and the nucleus. Eventually, the contractile elements are replaced with connective tissues. To conclude, the dystrophic gene is transcribed into a structural protein abnormality which directly or indirectly results in membrane "leakiness". The establishment of an abnormal ionic equilibrium across the membrane, especially that of Na^+, constitutes the earliest detectable pathophysiology in mediating weakness and necrosis of dystrophic myofibers.

Using a normal/dystrophic parabiotic mice model, it was demonstrated that the dystrophic nervous system was normal in its ability to form new innervation, to induce fiber type differentiation, to bring to maturity, and to maintain the structure and function of a normal muscle [28-30]. Without such knowledge, it would be imprudent to attempt strengthening dystrophic muscles with normal myogenic cell transfer.

MUSCLE TRANSPLANTATION AND REGENERATION

Normal Regenerates

Studies of mammalian muscle transplantation and regeneration in the seventies and earlier were confined to techniques of grafting whole muscles [31-35] and implanting muscle minces [36-39]. Grafting mature muscle suffers from slow reinnervation and revascularization of the inner myofibers that inevitably degenerated. Mincing traumatizes myofibers, producing pyknotic myonuclei, fragmented sarcolemma, denuded basement membranes, and degenerating cellular organelles [40-43]. Both procedures of muscle transplantation yield reduced function of the regenerates when compared to intact control muscles.

Satellite Cells

Satellite cells are the major source of myoblasts during regeneration [44,45]. The undifferentiated satellite cells are mobilized upon muscle injury to multiply and become myoblasts, that eventually fuse to form myotubes. It is estimated that 11% of all nuclei within the external lamina of normal muscle fibers in the gastrocnemius and soleus muscles of the rat belonged to satellite cells, and that only 6% of the nuclei remained viable 8 to 10 h after mincing. This 6% fraction would undergo mitosis before fusion [41,42]. When expressed as a percentage of the total number of myonuclei in a muscle fiber, satellite cell contribution becomes less with age [46].

Dystrophic Regenerates

The soleus of the C57BL/6J-dy2J dy2J dystrophic mouse is similar in number of muscle fibers to the soleus of a normal littermate at birth [47]. Muscle fiber loss begins at the second week after birth, and reaches a plateau of 50% loss at the fifteenth week. A similar percentage of fiber loss was observed from the third to the sixth postnatal week in 129/ReJ-dydy dystrophic mice [48,49]. Since there is no mechanism that can completely prevent muscle degeneration, and since dystrophic muscles exhibit poor regenerative capability [50,51], muscle weakness can best be reduced by replenishing the muscle fiber loss with genotypically normal cells.

Grafting mature muscles has not been successful. Because of the large size of a mature muscle graft, the deeper fibers in the muscle core are subjected to hypoxia. They often degenerate before becoming reinnnervated and revascularized [31-35]. Transplanting minced muscle fragments may overcome hypoxia and facilitate reinnervation [36]. However, mincing is such a traumatic procedure that the regenerated muscle always develops fewer fibers and contractile ability is greatly reduced [50,52].

Various factors contribute to account for the reduced capability of dystrophic muscles to regenerate. At the initiation of regeneration, myoblasts align themselves along the basement membrane and undergo mitosis [40,51]. Unlike crush lesions, which cause no disruption of the basement membrane, muscle minces cause basement membranes to fragment [41,42]. Such fragmentation destroys the scaffold for orderly cell replacement [54] and reduces the chances for complete regeneration. This explains why, even in normal animals, regenerated muscles from muscle minces cannot produce as much tension as unoperated muscles [52]. In the regeneration of dystrophic muscle minces, the problem is further complicated by a primary membrane defect such that the plasma membrane may not become properly regenerated after mincing. This deficiency would cause an infiltration of collagen and the deposition of connective tissues [40,53,55] that impedes innervation, thus aborting the maturation of the myotubes [51,55]. Failure to replace the damaged basement membrane may also result in a reduction in the number of regenerating myoblasts, because mitosis will stop as soon as the basement membrane is populated [40,53,55]. It was demonstrated that there was an increase in the number of satellite cells in muscles of patients with Duchenne muscular dystrophy compared to that in normal controls [56].

In regenerating dystrophic muscles, the regenerative capability is likely to be limited by the failure of basement and plasma membrane reformation, by the infiltration of collagen, and by the number of satellite cells that are present immediately after mincing. Another parameter that is important in the regeneration of muscle is muscle activity. Innervated young muscle fibers require constant active and passive muscle activities for normal differentiation and morphogenesis [40]. Such activities are not to be found in the regenerating dystrophic muscles, because neighboring muscles have already been undergoing degeneration, and the newly established motor endplates in the regenerate do not function as efficiently as normal.

Early muscle transplant studies in murine dystrophy research were designed to test whether muscular dystrophy is neurogenic or myogenic [57-61]. These studies always specified removal of a host muscle, which was then reimplanted or replaced with a foreign muscle. The procedure introduces two deficiencies. First, it replaces a functioning muscle with one which is nonfunctioning until it becomes reinnervated, thereby upsetting the balance in the activities of synergistic and antagonistic muscles of the host [62-65]. Such imbalance of muscle activity may eventually be reflected in the regenerative condition of the transplanted muscle [66-69]. Second, whenever the host nerve is cut, fewer than 50% of its fibers will survive to reinnervate [70-72]. This is especially significant in the dystrophic soleus nerve, which exhibits spontaneous reduction in the number of motor axons [73]. In designing a system to reduce muscle weakness, it is obviously advantageous not to remove the host muscle, so as to allow uninterrupted nerve and muscle function.

GENE TRANSFER

Dystrophyc Genes

The development of recombinant DNA, DNA sequencing and gene transfer techniques [74-77] hold the implicit promise to correct genetic diseases by correcting the abnormal gene itself. Through positional cloning [78], the dystrophin gene, whose absence or alteration results in Duchenne and Becker muscular dystrophies, has been located on chromosome Xp21 and sequenced [8,9,79,80]. Its 79 exons and introns span 2.5 megabases of genomic DNA and encode a 14 kilobase mRNA. The latter translates the missing protein dystrophin [7,80]. The gene responsible for myotonic dystrophy has also been isolated [81-83]. In addition, genes responsible for facioscapulohumeral dystrophy [84], limb-girdle dystrophy [85,86] and Emery Dreifuss muscular dystrophy [87] have been located on specific chromosomes through linkage analyses.

The above knowledge allows diagnosis at the molecular genetics level, which is especially significant in the differential diagnosis of Duchenne vs Becker muscular dystrophy [80,88]. It also offers advantages in prenatal counseling and carrier detection. Gene manipulation and transferal, being explored in animals, has sparked much hope for cure or treatment for the dystrophies. It is worthwhile to fully understand the conceptual approach, the evidence, the potentials and limitations of these approaches.

Dystrophin

Expression of the large dystrophin gene involves at least five promoters with very complex transcriptional and splicing control [89]. Dystrophin is a cytoskeletal membrane protein similar to β-spectrin and α-actinin [7,90]. It consists of 3685 amino acids with a molecular weight of 427 kilodaltons (kD), and folds into distinct structural domains: the amino (N) terminuus the "rod region" and the carboxy (C) terminus [89].

Dystrophin comprises about 0.001% of total protein in normal human muscles [7]. It is mainly localized on the inner surface of the plasma membrane. A different isoform is found in brain. Dystrophin is absent in DMD, and is reduced or altered in BMD [80,91]. Exceptions have been reported. Two BMD patients have been found without dystrophin [92], and a DMD patient shows a dystrophin phenotype indistinguishable from normal [93]. Overall, there is a correlation of deletion type (DMD vs. BMD), severity of the disease and the quantity and quality of dystrophin [89,93]. This is especially true if DMD and BMD are considered as one disease entity, the Xp21 myopathy.

Dystrophin is a large structural protein in close association to glycoproteins in the plasma membrane of normal myotubes or myofibers. The dystrophin/glycoproteins complex provides support to the cell membrane cytoskeleton.

Unlike the mdx mice, dystrophic mice (strain 129, Strain C57BL/6J-dy2Jdy2J) showed the presence of dystrophin in the plasma membrane of their skeletal muscles. The genetic defects of these mice are manifested in the absence of laminin, a membrane protein defect which is also found in Severe Childhood Autosomal Recessive Muscular Dystrophy (SCARMD). Their muscle degeneration parallels DMD in spite of the presence of dystrophin. The mdx mice exhibit essentially normal muscle function and lifespan in spite of the absence of dystrophin.

Whereas dystrophin serves as a good genetic/biochemical marker, more pertinent is the technical question of how to replace dystrophin. "The ultimate goal of rational therapy of Duchenne muscular dystrophy is clear: to replace dystrophin within muscle fibers" [94].

Dystrophin Up-Regulation

Up-regulation of dystrophin has been proposed as a therapeutic strategy for DMD. The incorporation of large structural protein(s) such as dystrophin into cell membranes has defied current technologies. Retroviral infection of mature myofibers with conjugated factor(s) to up-regulate dystrophin production seems inadequate in view of low efficiency, high risk and instability of transduction.

Contrary to common belief, dystrophin replacement constitutes only a part of the treatment. It has already been demonstrated using MTT in mdx mice [95-97] and in humans [98-105]. Since DMD pathology is one of muscle degeneration and weakness, structural and especially functional improvements have to be the primary concerns. Expression of a foreign gene requires appropriate integration and regulation involving numerous cofactors, many of which are transient during embryonic development. This is especially true in the deposit of structural proteins such as dystrophin, rather than in the secretion of enzymes or hormones.

Genes only transmit biological characteristics but are not primary functioning units like cells of the body. Like drug therapy, dystrophin up-regulation cannot replenish degenerated cells. At best, it can only repair degenerating cells. In a 12-year-old DMD boy in which over 70% of the muscle cells have been lost from the quadriceps, it is unlikely that dystrophin replacement in the remaining cells alone will bring forth a cure or a treatment, whatever the delivery system of dystrophin may be.

Plasmid Injection

When plasmid DNA of the dystrophin gene is injected intramuscularly into dystrophin-deficient mdx mice, dystrophin is found seven days later in about 1% of the myofibers [106-108]. Retroviral-mediated transfer increases the efficiency to 6% [109], whereas adenovirus-mediated transfer boosts it to 50% [110]. The authors conclude that there is a direct correlation between the level of muscle fibers expressing recombinant dystrophin and the level of muscle fibers with peripheral nuclei, indicating an improvement in muscle pathology [106,108].

Only a very small number of muscle fibers show dystrophin, and central nucleation is the only parameter used in monitoring normality in muscle pathology. Mature mdx mice are not totally devoid of dystrophin. Their muscles often contain over 1% of dystrophin-positive fibers. Since mdx mice do not exhibit muscle weakness and shortened life expectancy, the dystrophic dog (GRMD) is a better animal model [111] to demonstrate the efficacy of plasmid injection in which dystrophin production, cell structure and muscle function can be monitored. To date, plasmid delivery into dystrophic animals has not led to clinical trial of humanmuscular dystrophy.

Based on transgenic mice studies [112], clinical trials on cystic fibrosis (CF) and on severe combined immunodeficiency (SCID) [113] using viral vector single gene transduction were attempted and met with limited success. Unlike CF and SCID whose genetic defects are mediated through enzymatic deficiencies, DMD is caused by a deficit of a structural protein rather than a regulatory protein.

While optimism soars as transgenes were expressed in skeletal myofibers [114,115] and cardiac cells [116,117], the mechanism of uptake of plasmid DNA was not known [115], and the efficiency of transduction was low. Plasmid injection, if it ever becomes a treatment for DMD or heart failure, would have to be administered before any major cell degeneration occurs.

Transfected Myoblast Transfer

This was the original approach proposed in gene manipulation toward DMD treatment [118]. The procedure consists of a) obtaining a muscle biopsy from the DMD patient, b) transducing a "seed" amount of satellite cells with the dystrophin gene, c) confirming the myogenicity of the transfected cells, d) proliferating the transduced myoblasts to an amount enough to produce beneficial effect and e) injecting the myoblasts into the patient.

Retroviral vectors have been used to transfer genes into rat and dog myoblasts in primary cultures under conditions that permit the transduced myoblasts to differentiate into myotubes and expressing the transferred genes [119]. Furthermore, mice injected with murine myoblasts that are transfected with human growth hormone (hGH) show significant levels of hGH in both muscle and serum that are stable for 3 months [120,121]. The transduced myoblast transfer for DMD is similar in approach to the study of adenosine deaminase (ADA) deficiency. In the latter, T cells from the patient were transduced with functional ADA genes and returned to the patient after expansion in the number of the transduced cells through cell culture [122].

How realistic is such an approach for DMD? When the recombinant human dystrophin gene is integrated stably into mouse myoblasts in culture, these cells express the gene and synthesize recombinant dystrophin protein of the correct size and appropriate antibody reactivity [123]. However, the precise mechanisms of gene integration, regulation and expression are not known (Table 1). Imagine a large DNA-retroviral conjugate traversing the myoblast cell membrane, its cytoskeleton and possibly the nuclear membrane. The myoblast has to remain physically undamaged. Oncogenes should not be turned on to produce tumors. A sufficient amount, e.g. 10^5, of such "seed" myoblasts will have to be produced with molecular manipulation, and then be cloned to produce 50 X 10^9 cells for the myoblast injection treatment, without any loss of myogenicity or any acquisition of tumorgenicity.

Table 1. Gene manipulation versus myoblast transfer in repairing DMD muscle fibers

Procedure	Gene manipulation	Myoblast transfer
Identify defective gene	achieved	bypass
Synthesize normal gene	achieved	bypass
Target gene to tissue	injection	injection
Target gene into cells	viruses	natural cell fusion
Integrate normal gene	rare, random	natural
Regulate normal gene	not achieved	natural
Express normal gene	rare, inconsistent	natural

(Reproduced with permission from Law et al; Cell Transplantation 1:235, 1992).

Unfortunately, delivering transduced autologous myoblasts to treat DMD muscles has encountered low efficiency and mutation in transduction [119-121], and will yield insufficient myogenic cells to provide for a whole body MTT [124]. The down-sized dystrophin gene is still at least five times too big for efficient viral vector transduction. It cannot perform exactly like the full-size gene. Viral vectors may revert to pathologic states and cause acute pneumonia as encounted in a clinical trial of CF using adenovirus mediated vector. Although the myoblast clones are histocompatible with the recipient, the dystrophin recombinant, being derived from a foreign gene, is foreign to the host immune system. This is a complicated, uncertain, and a very expensive way to obtain histocompatible normal myoblasts, and does not offer any advantage over normal MTT.

With this approach, myoblast transfer is still part of the therapy. Adenovirus vector in high titre [10^{10} pfu/ml or above] can efficiently transduce immature muscle cells but not mature nuscle fibers in vivo [125]. Every step of the therapy will have to be custom tailored for each patient for histocompatibility. Even if such a procedure does become available many years from now, the technology will be too late to help many.

Arterial delivery of genetically transformed myoblasts into rat skeletal muscles has been reported [126]. It is difficult to reconcile the survival of myoblasts in the blood stream where macrophages and leukocytes abound. If these myoblasts indeed survive, they will undoubtedly divide in the rich milieu of the blood stream and fuse when they reach confluence in the capillaries. The latter will introduce risks of thrombi formation, possibly leading to pulmonary embolism. The recombinant DNA research has not provided a cure or treatment for DMD [124,127].

The success in transgenic mouse production, though rare, does indicate that gene manipulation can be effective in phenotype transformation when applied in embryos [128]. It is through manipulating the embryo that the normal gene may possibly transfect all cells of the adult to achieve a cure. However, such approach in humans would seem impractical for ethical, religious and technical reasons.

Dystrophin-Associated Glycoproteins (DAGs)

Dystrophin exists in a large oligomeric complex with the transmembrane glycoproteins of 35 kD (35-DAG), 43 kD (43-DAG) and 50 kD (50-DAG), an extracellular glycoprotein of 156 kD (156-DAG) and a cytoskeletal protein of 59 kD (59-DAG) [129-132]. The complex links the subsarcolemmal cytoskeleton to the extracellular matrix through the binding of 156-DAG to laminin. The DAGs are reduced in muscles of DMD [133], Fukuyama congenital muscular dystrophy [134], mdx [135] and the cardiomyopathic hamster [136]. Absence of DAGs can cause degeneration by themselves [133].

Hypothetically, the absence of dystrophin causes a disruption of the sarcolemmal linkage, with the loss of DAGs, especially during muscle contraction, and results in cell necrosis and muscle weakness in DMD [133]. As more myogenic transcription factors are discovered and their functions defined [137,138], it is hoped that those regulating the expression of dystrophin and DAGs will soon be unveiled.

Perspectives

Human gene therapy is a procedure that was used in attempts to treat genetic diseases such as cystic fibrosis (CF) and severe combined immunodeficiency (SCID). Human genetic engineering raises unique safety, social and ethical concerns [139]. Unlike CF and SCID whose defects through life are single enzymatic deficiencies, DMD symptoms are caused by a deficit of several structural proteins rather than a single regulatory protein. This latter difference plays an important role in deciding whether single gene manipulation is the direction we should take in developing treatment for DMD and the other muscular dystrophies.

As mentioned earlier, expression of a foreign gene requires appropriate integration and regulation involving polygenomic interaction and numerous cofactors, many of which are transient and unknown during embryonic development. This is especially true in the deposit of structural proteins such as dystrophin than in the secretion of enzymes such as adenosine deaminase (ADA). Since muscle cells of DMD boys lack not only dystrophin but dystrophin-related proteins and glycoproteins [133,140], and since the absence of these latter proteins can cause dystrophy by themselves [133,140], single gene replacement will not be effective in repairing the defective cells except for the very young patients in whom cell degeneration has not begun. There is no better method than MTT to replace all of these proteins through natural integration of the normal genome. Thus, MTT is not a stop-gap but conceptually the best possible treatment for the current DMD population.

Whereas single gene manipulation still harbors many unknowns [141], its success toward treatment of muscular dystrophy has been very limited. Even when fully developed, the procedure can only repair degenerating cells but cannot replenish degenerated cells. Gene therapists need to be cognizant of the fact that multiple gene integration will be necessary to repair myofibers of the current DMD population, and that these clinical trials are still many years away. The sooner researchers acknowledge the limitations of gene manipulation [124,126,141,142], the sooner will research efforts be focused toward developing myoblast transfer as the therapy for muscular dystrophy.

Myoblast Transfer

The terms "Myoblast Transfer" and "Myoblast Transfer Therapy" (MTT) were coined in a workshop held in Perth, Western Australia on February 20-22, 1989 [143]. Within four months, the First International Conference on Myoblast Transfer Therapy was held in New York City on June 10-12, 1989 [144]. In both meetings, international experts concluded that MTT was the most logical approach in the development of muscle disease treatment. In addition to continued animal research on MTT, small-scale clinical trials were initiated to determine the safety and efficacy of the procedure in humans. MTT thus appeared as a breakthrough with a quantum leap from animal experimentation into human study. Until now, the term "MTT" has been used in the scientific literature interchangeably for animal and human studies. However, in human studies, a more appropriate term is "Human Myoblast Genome Therapy" or "HMGT" because of the concomitant cell therapy and genome therapy procedure as explained below.

What is MTT or HMGT?

MTT or HMGT is a platform technology of cell transplantation, nuclear transfer, and tissue engineering developed to treat diseases associated with muscle degeneration and weakness. It is also used to enhance normal or near-normal physical conditions.

Myoblasts are differentiated, immature cells destined to become muscles. Myoblasts cultured from muscle biopsy survive, develop and function to revitalize degenerative muscles after transplantation.

The myoblast transplant procedure incorporates cell therapy and genome therapy concomitantly. Transplant injury activates regeneration of the host myofibers that fuse with the injected myoblasts, sharing their nuclei in a common gene pool of the myofiber synctium. Through nuclear transfer and complementation, the normal human genome can be transferred into muscle cells of genetically-ill patients to achieve phenotype *repair*. Myoblasts are safe and efficient gene transfer vehicles endogenous to muscles. Since muscles constitute 50% of the human body, extremely precise dosing of secreted biologics can be achieved from transduced myoblasts implanted. In addition, myoblasts fuse among themselves to form new myofibres to *replenish* those that underwent degeneration. The procedure leads to the formation of a genetically mosaic muscle (Figure 3).

Only 2-month cyclosporine immunosuppression is sufficient to prevent allograft rejection because myofibres do not express MHC-1 antigens. Only allografts instead of autografts can be used in the treatment of genetic disorders because myoblasts of the genetically-ill patients carry the same genetic defect(s) (Table 2). Allografts also have advantage over autografts when transduced myoblasts are targeted to secret foreign therapeutic protein(s).

The procedure involves isolation and culturing of satellite cells derived from muscle biopsies of genetically normal donors. It is customary to refer to myoblast reserves in adult muscles as satellite cells, and satellite cells in culture as myoblasts. Cell culture mass-produces the myoblasts and removes the antigenic leukocytes, adipocytes and fibroblasts. These donor myoblasts are then injected or surgically implanted into a number of foci in the degenerative muscles where host satellite cells and regenerating myofibers are abound.

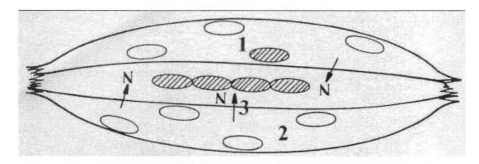

Figure 3. Injection of normal myoblasts into the dystrophic mouse muscle resulted in the formation of a mosaic muscle with normal, dystrophic, and mosaic myofibers. Two genetic complementation mechanisms were shown to alleviate muscle weakness: (1) normal gene product, N, in the mosaic fibers suppresses dystrophy expression; (2) developing normal fibers progressively replaced degenerative fibers. A third possibility (3), normal fibers supplying a diffusible "corrective factor" N to supplement neighboring dystrophic fibers, was not examined. Open ovals, normal nuclei; shaded ovals, dystrophic nuclei. (Reproduced with permission from Law et al. 1988.)

Table 2. Autograft versus allograft for the regenerative heart

	AUTOGRAFT	ALLOGRAFT	
PROS	No immunosuppression	2-mo immunosuppression	CONS
CONS	Cell culture takes 1-mo	Good cells readily available	PROS
	Graft delay ⟶ scar	Grafting within 12 hr ⇸ scar	
	Elderly cells less regenerative	Young cells rejuvenate	
	High QA/QC costs for each individual graft	Low QA/QC costs for 50 grafts at a time	
	Host limitation	Unlimited supply	
	Infected/mutated host tissues may contaminate system	Patients with infections and genetic diseases can be treated	

The idea of using myoblasts as donor cells in MTT/HMGT is to provide the genetic blueprint to be activated through the regeneration process. Although mammalian skeletal muscles are capable of regeneration, there are not enough satellite cells to fully compensate for major muscle damage in the body. Furthermore, muscle regeneration is abortive in DMD. Treatment or cure involving single gene manipulation will have to be conducted on young patients or even fetuses rather than on older individuals, whose muscle cells have significantly degenerated. This differs from MTT/HMGT which *replenishes* lost cells and *repairs* degenerating cells.

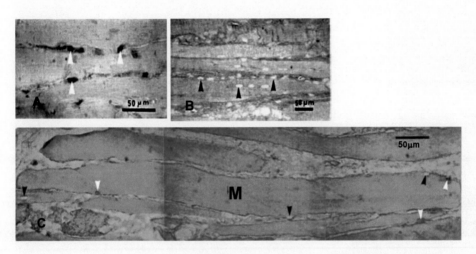

Figure 4. Immunocytochemical localization of donor (stained, white arrowheads) and host (unstained, dark arrowheads) nuclei in longitudinal muscle sections. A and B are normal and dystrophic controls, respectively. C is from a dystrophic muscle 18 months after normal myoblast injection. A mosaic fiber (M) is demonstrated by the presence of both stained and unstained nuclei. (Reproduced with permission from Law et al. 1990.)

How MTT/HMGT Works?

Dystrophic cells degenerate because they lack a normal gene. Such degeneration can be prevented by incorporation of full complements of normal genes through cell fusion with donor myoblasts [145-148]. Cell fusion is a spontaneous occurrence during myogenesis [149] and muscle regeneration [150,151]. When normal myoblasts are transferred into a regenerating dystrophic muscle as in MTT/HMGT, the donor cells fuse spontaneously with the host satellite cells and/or the host myofibers themselves to form mosaic fibers, sharing their normal genes to produce normal cell phenotype (Figure 4). Furthermore, donor myoblasts fuse among themselves to form myotubes that develop into normal myofibers (Figures 5, 6C, 6D). These normal myofibers progressively replace the degenerative host fibers. MTT/HMGT thus repairs degenerating cells and replenishes lost cells.

It does not matter which gene is abnormal or which protein is missing; MTT/HMGT has the potential to prevent genetically abnormal muscle cells from degenerating, regardless of the genetic defect. Through genetic complementation, the inserted normal genes encode one or more missing protein(s) (or factors) to supplement the metabolism or development of the heterokaryons, thereby sustaining the normal integrity of these genetically transformed cells. In this respect, MTT/HMGT differs from bone marrow grafting which is based strictly on the replacement strategy where cell fusion and genetic complementation do not occur. MTT/HMGT is the first therapy that has demonstrated significant improvement in cell genetics and phenotypes of live mammals [145-148].

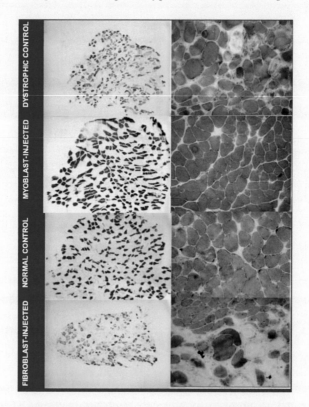

Figure 5. When compared with contralateral controls 6 months postoperatively, myoblast-injected dystrophic solei exhibited greater cross-sectional area and total fiber number. They contained more normal appearing and less abnormal-appearing fibers. Injection of about 10^6 fibroblasts as a control for cell type resulted in less absolute number of fibers, higher percentage of abnormal fibers, and more connective tissues in test dystrophic solei. (Reproduced with permission from Law et al. 1988).

The MTT/HMGT concept is based on previous work on muscle development, regeneration, transplantation, reinnervation, and genetic complementation. Because skeletal muscles of all mammals behave similarly in these situations, MTT/HMGT should have application to all mammalian muscle diseases including those of humans. Augmentation in muscle size, shape, consistency and force are not only therapeutic for muscle diseases, but should also be useful in disease prevention and enhancement of physical conditions.

Origin of MTT/HMGT

It is not possible to turn an already dystrophic individual into a totally normal one. The best alternative is to transform the dystrophic individual to become similar to the X-linked carrier in order to achieve normal or near-normal function. According to the Lyon hypothesis [152], random inactivation of one or the other X-chromosome can occur in any nucleus throughout the body of a Duchenne female carrier; individual muscle fibers would therefore contain mixtures of normal and dystrophic nuclei similar to the mosaic fibers produced by injecting normal myoblasts into dy2Jdy2J muscles (Figure 4). The mosaic fibers exhibit normal phenotype, presumably due to metabolic or developmental complementation as a result of sharing the normal nuclei and therefore the normal genes. In addition, muscles of chimeric mice containing fibers of normal, dystrophic and mosaic genotypes exhibit normal function [153]. It thus appears that the logical and practical approach to reverse the expression of dystrophy in muscles of adult animals is to induce genetic mosaicism through the incorporation of the normal nuclei. This can be accomplished by transplantation of myogenic cells.

Neural Hypothesis of Muscular Dystrophy

A serious consideration in these muscle transplant studies is whether the nervous system of dystrophic individuals will support normal muscle development. The approach of muscle transplant would not be effective if the dystrophic nervous system induces degenerative changes in the regenerate. In the parabiotic mice study of Law et al [28], in which a "fast" dystrophic nerve was transposed onto a "slow" normal muscle, it was demonstrated that the dystrophic nerve is normal in its ability to form synapses, to induce fiber-type differentiation, to bring fibers to maturity, and to maintain the structural and functional integrity of normal muscle fibers. This parabiotic mice study also provides strong evidence against a neural etiology of murine dystrophy.

A study often cited to support the neural hypothesis is the chimeric mouse study of Peterson11 who concludes that "extramuscular factors must be implicated in muscular dystrophy". This conclusion is based on Peterson's argument that a small population of normal nuclei could not have prevented dystrophic pathology in the chimeric muscles that showed normal histology and isometric twitch tensions. However, such argument contradicts Peterson's later claim that "only a very small proportion of genotypically normal myonuclei were required for expression of an apparently normal phenotype [154]. In view of the parabiotic mice studies [28, 29, 30] it would appear that muscle degeneration in the dystrophic mice is not primarily caused by neurotrophic deficiency or by a lack of myelin as previously claimed by others [155-158]. Whereas both nerve and muscle cells are susceptible to the dystrophic gene action, muscle cells are more vulnerable to degeneration because of their contractile activity [27,30].

Animal Models

The dystrophic mice (129 ReJ-dydy and C57BL/6J-dy2Jdy2J strains) are excellent models of hereditary muscle degeneration and weakening [22,23,159] and are most studied. The autosomal recessive inheritance is manifested as progressive cell degeneration mainly in muscle and, to a minor extent, in nerve [148,73]. The crippling pathology, associated with significant muscle weakness, is similar to most forms of human dystrophies. In addition, these mice bear a close resemblance to DMD boys and children with SCARMD in that premature death occurs as a result of respiratory failure. Another animal model is the mdx mouse which does not show functional deficit or premature death [160-163]. Its muscle pathology does not show fiber splitting, phagocytic necrosis, and infiltration of fat and connective tissues, all of which are diagnostic features of dystrophy. Muscle pathology of mdx includes a brief period of central nucleation which is often interpreted as necrosis but may also represent delayed maturation or regeneration of the myofibers. Nevertheless, many consider mdx as a better genetic model of DMD because both diseases are X-linked recessive and both lack dystrophin.

The more ideal model for DMD is the dystrophic dog which shows a similar mode of inheritance, severe progressive muscle degeneration and weakness, and a lack of dystrophin [164,165]. The dystrophic dog offers advantage over the dy2Jdy2J mouse for MTT/HMGT research because, as in human, its larger muscles provide a more realistic challenge to the culturing and placement of donor myoblasts. In addition, dystrophin can be used as a biochemical marker to demonstrate successful engrafting in the dystrophic dog but not in the dy2Jdy2J mouse, since muscles of the mouse produce dystrophin [166].

Cell Therapy VS Gene Therapy

It is erroneous to believe that MTT/HMGT stems from the molecular studies of dystrophic genes or the proteins they encoded. The original testing of the MTT/HMGT idea was published in 1978 [150], and the complete cloning of the DMD gene did not appear until 1987 [9]. MTT/HMGT is developed according to the knowledge of genetic complementation which circumvents the time-consuming and expensive processes of abnormal gene identification, therapeutic gene synthesis, tissue targeting, gene integration, regulation, and expression that are not fully understood. The spontaneous cell fusion process inherent in myogenesis and muscle regeneration is utilized to incorporate the normal nuclei into dystrophic muscle cells. Since the fusion process is a natural occurrence, there should not be any problem with specificities of integration, complementation, regulation, and expression of the normal genes inserted. It is not necessary to know which gene(s) is responsible for the defect. Furthermore, the injection of normal myoblasts directly into the dystrophic muscle eliminates the uncertainty of tissue targeting with gene therapy. By virtue of incorporation of full complements of normal genes into genetically abnormal cells to achieve repair, MTT/HMGT is a gene therapy, or better still, a genome therapy.

The essence of MTT/HMGT is that it does not matter which gene or protein is missing. Through the incorporation of donor myonuclei, dystrophic cells are replenished with full complements of normal genes that are allowed to express and interact spontaneously. This differs from gene therapy in which a single gene is manipulated into the abnormal cell where cofactors essential for the regulation and expression of the gene may no longer be present at the developmental stage of the cell.

MTT/HMGT is the first cell therapy in which genetic engineering has demonstrated significant success in mammals. The ability to produce genotypic and phenotypic improvement through incorporation of the normal genes opens new avenues for other genetic diseases. Since many genetic diseases are fatal, the less time-consuming genetic complementation approach should be the method of choice in the development of treatments.

Development of MTT/HMGT

The original idea of MTT/HMGT, and experiments testing MTT/HMGT, were first published by Law in 1978 [50]. A deliberate attempt was made in adult dystrophic mice to produce mosaic muscles containing normal, dystrophic and mosaic myofibers from the regenerates of normal and dystrophic minced muscle mixes. The mince and mix procedure was designed to provide an environment for the intermingling and fusion of normal and dystrophic satellite cells. These muscle regenerates produced greater twitch and tetanus tensions and more normal appearing cell structure than control regenerates of minced dystrophic muscles. It was concluded that the introduction of cell contents of normal genotype into dystrophic muscles could improve the function of the latter.

The result contradicts the study of Partridge and Sloper who concluded, in transplanting normal minced muscles into normal hosts, that little or none of the regenerates was of donor origin [167]. These latter authors suggested the possibility of introducing, by a systemic route, normal muscle nuclei into diseased muscle fibers. Attractive though it seemed, this latter idea would not have been in agreement with knowledge of myoblast characteristics. Apart from the risks of having the circulatory system congested with rapidly dividing myoblasts, capillaries ruptured by growing myotubes, and severe host immune response against myoblast surface antigens, it is doubtful if the myoblasts are small enough to exit the wall of the capillaries. In the Anglo-French Cellular Therapy Meeting held in Cambridge, England on April 2-3, 1990, Kornegay reported the absence of a beneficial effect after intraarterial injection of donor myoblasts into two dystrophic golden retriever dogs. There was no evidence that any component of the donor myoblasts entered the skeletal muscles.

Concurrent with Law's 1978 publication on normal/dystrophic transplant was that of Partridge, Grounds, and Sloper, which described fusion between host and donor myogenic cells of normal genotypes using skeletal muscle grafts [168]. Contrary to what these authors previously published, they now claimed satellite cells did survive and develop in normal host muscles. Although the study did not involve dystrophic animals, the author inferred that MTT was a distinct development with potential applicability to hereditary myopathies.

Law's subsequent experiments were designed to bypass the trauma introduced by mincing. Interruption of the connections of nerve, blood, and tendon had to be avoided. A new muscle transplant method had to be developed. Knowing that the dystrophic nerve would support normal muscle development [28,30], Law grafted intact muscles of newborn normal mice into recipient soleus muscles of dsytrophic mice at the first clinical sign of dystrophy [169]. Results obtained 6 months after the grafting indicated that muscle fibers of the grafts survived, developed, and functioned in the dystrophic environment The regenerates had larger cross-sectional areas and more muscle fibers than the contralateral dystrophic solei. *That was the first study in muscular dystrophy research to have successfully improved the twitch tension of an adult dystrophic muscle to that of a normal.*

Grafting newborn muscle in animal is an innovative method of muscle transplant. The method eliminates tendon damage, overcomes hypoxia, and facilitates reinnervation and revascularization of the grafted muscle fibers, thus promoting the survival and development of the characteristics of the donor muscle [169]. The result achieved is superior to that obtained from mature muscle grafts or from minced muscle transplants. In addition to treatment of recessive myopathies of autosomal dominant inheritance, where rescue relies more on replenishing lost cells rather than on nuclear complementation after mosaic fiber formation. *A corollary to MTT/HMGT is to allow donor myoblasts to fuse in culture and to transplant the resulting myotubes that form the major component in newborn muscles.* By 1979, the concept of replenishing lost cells and repairing degenerative cells through the production of muscle mosaicism using MTT/HMGT was firmly established [169]. In the same year, it was established that myoblasts cultured from muscle biopsies of adult normal rats could survive and develop in the original donor after implantation [170].

Nevertheless, grafting newborn muscles has limited applicability in humans, because human newborn muscles are too large for rapid reinnervation and revascularization. There are also the ethical considerations. It is necessary to develop the myoblast transplant techniques.

A convenient way to obtain myoblasts in mice is through dissection of *limb-bud mesenchyme* of embryos. The first successful implantation of normal myoblasts into dystrophic mouse muscles was published by Law in 1982 [171]. Mesenchymal tissue rich in myoblasts (about 80% myoblasts, 20% fibreblasts) was dissected from limb-buds of day-12 normal mouse embryos. It was surgically implanted into the right solei of 20-day-old normal or dystrophic C56BL6J-dy2Jdy2J mice. Host and donors were histocompatible. Unoperated left solei served as controls. Sham control solei receiving similar surgical treatment but no mesenchyme transplant did not differ from contralateral, unoperated solei. This argues against the possibility that trauma to dystrophic muscles or their innervation could induce long-term improvement in muscle structure and function as claimed by Ontell [172].

Six to seven months postoperatively, the myoblast-implanted solei exhibited greater cross-sectional area, total fiber number, and twitch and tetanus tensions than their contralateral controls. Test dystrophic solei contained more normal-appearing and less abnormal-appearing fibers than their controls. The results indicate that such transplantation improves the structure and function of the dystrophic muscles [184]. In this study, the donor cells were not cultured before implantation, and recipient muscles were not subjected to denervation.

Meanwhile, the laboratory of Sloper and Partridge continued to explore factors that affected the incorporation and fusion of allogeneic muscle precursor cells in vivo [173]. Their studies involved only normal but not dystrophic mice. The implants consisted of either minced muscle mixes or newborn muscles disaggregated by trypsin and pargestin [174-176]. In both cases, they were implanted for two months or less in muscle compartments where the host muscles were removed. Such experimental design introduced denervation, devascularization and tendon detachment. It did not allow the muscle regenerates enough time to develop good structure or function. The authors demonstrated the survival and development of donor cells in the host muscles, using electrophoretic analyses of glucose phosphate isomerases (GPI), the genetic markers to identify hosts vs. donor cells.

Partridge's laboratory did not report implantation into abnormal muscles until 1988, when they employed the ICR/IAn mice as hosts [176]. These mice exhibited a mild glycogen-storage myopathy associated with a genetic lack of muscle phosphorylase kinase (PhK), but no significant structural or functional abnormality was apparent [177]. Enzymic disaggregation of neonatal muscle was employed to produce muscle precursor cells, resulting in only a small proportion of myogenic cells in the injected suspension. Although there have been frequent claims of supplying normal muscle precursor cells to alleviate hereditary myopathies by these authors, no evidence of any structural or functional improvement after transplantation was presented. In fact, these authors have not reported working with any dystrophic muscles having structural and functional deficits at all.

1988 witnessed the explosive development of MTT/HMGT following two significant publications in June by Law et al. [145,146]. In the first study, primary myoblast cultures from limb-bud explants of normal mouse embryos were injected into the soleus muscles of histocompatible dystrophic hosts [145]. In the second study, clones of normal myoblasts were injected into the leg and intercostal muscles on both sides of histoincompatible hosts with cyclosporine-A (CsA) as host immunosuppressant [146]. In both cases, donor myoblasts fused among themselves, developing into normal myofibers that progressively replaced the degenerated fibers. They also fused with dystrophic host myogenic cells to form mosaic myofibers of normal phenotype [145-148]. These two mechanisms of genetic complementation were shown to be responsible for significant improvement in muscle genetics, structure, function and animal behavior of the test dystrophic mice. In later reports, prolongation of the life-spans of the myoblast-injected dystrophic mice was demonstrated [147,148].

Morgan et al. reported the synthesis of trace amounts of PhK in about 5% of the myoblast-injected muscles of the PhK-deficient mice [176]. Seven months later, Partridge et al. reported the conversion of mdx myofibers from dystrophin-negative to -positive 20 to 50 days after injections of normal myoblasts [96]. The authors claimed rescue of the host fibers from their biochemical defect. The study demonstrates biochemical improvement in the mdx mouse model, an additional evidence to confirm the efficacy of MTT/HMGT as previously reported by Law et al. who had demonstrated improved muscle cell genetics and structure, strength, mobility, general well-being, and longevity of the dy2Jdy2J mice [50,145,148,169,171]. Karpati et al. provided further confirmation that dystrophin is expressed in mdx myofibers after MTT [97].

MYOBLAST TRANSFER IMPROVES MUSCLE GENETICS/BIOCHEMISTRY/STRUCTURE/FUNCTION AND NORMALIZES THE BEHAVIOR AND LIFE SPAN OF DYSTROPHIC MICE

We shall now examine the experimental results from animal studies that lead to MTT/HMGT clinical trials in humans. All of the developmental work was published by essentially two research teams whose approaches were disparate but complementary. While Law and associates were demonstrating the safety and efficacy of transferring normal myogenic cells into the dy2Jdy2J dystrophic mice, Partridge and associates were examining the developmental fate of donor cells in normal mice.

This was at a time when neither the golden retriever muscular dystrophy (GRMD) nor the xmd canine dystrophy was widely known or available [164,165]. Indeed, most of what can be done in the dog can be done in half the time and at a fraction of the cost in the mouse. Although GRMD and xmd are excellent models for testing potential treatments, they are available to a few chosen laboratories that, because of technical deficiencies, have not produced any convincing experimental results with MTT [178].

It was not until 1989 that study of MTT on mdx mice was first published [96,97]. The majority of evidence in support of MTT/HMGT efficacy is derived from previous studies using the dy2Jdy2J mice [50,145-148,169,171].

Central to MTT/HMGT is the correlation of genetic and phenotypic improvement at the cellular and at the whole muscle levels. Such correlation has to be derived from demonstrations that in fact there are genotypic and phenotypic improvements. These studies play an essential role in the elucidation of the mechanisms by which MTT/HMGT exerts its beneficial effects [50,145-148,169,171].

Genetic Improvement

Isozymes of glucose-6-phosphate isomerase (GPI) have been used as genetic markers [179-181] to quantify myonuclear genotypes of mice. Initially the procedure was used to determine the genotypic constitution in muscles and other tissues of chimeric [182,153] mice. Eventually it was adopted for myoblast transfer studies because of the persistence of the GPI isozymes within individual cells throughout the whole life of the animal [145-148,183].

Each cell expresses the isoform(s) which is specific to the genes encoding GPI, regardless of whether the latter is of donor or host origin. For example, Watt et al. implanted myogenic cells of the 129/ReJ mouse, which is homozygous for the GPI-1a allele, into muscles of either C57BL/6J or ICR/IAn hosts that are homozygous for the GPI-1b allele [183]. Grafts of the muscle precursor cells were found to have survived and developed in the host muscles as demonstrated by the presence of the parental isozymes GPI-1AA, GPI-1BB in gel electrophoresis of whole muscles. In addition, the presence of the hybrid isozyme GPI-1AB indicated fusion between host and donor cells in about 10% of the host muscles examined. Because the host mice selected exhibit normal genotypes and normal motor function, it is impossible to determine if there was any phenotypic improvement. The study does demonstrate that myogenic cell implantation allows the introduction of normal genome into normal muscles at the cellular and at the whole muscle level. This study provides support and confirmation to the mechanisms responsible for the structural and functional improvement observed after myogenic cell transfer into the dy2Jdy2J mice [50,169,171].

Genetic improvement of dystrophic muscles appeared in publication in 1988, when Law et al. reported that normal myoblast injections provided genetic treatment for murine (dy2Jdy2J) dystrophy. Cultured myoblasts (10^6) from genetically normal mouse embryos were injected into the right soleus of 20-day-old normal or dystrophic mice. Hosts and donors were histocompatible but exhibited different genotype markers. Donor cells produced GPI-1CC. Host cells produced GPI-1BB.

The GPI-1c allele codes for an isozyme of greater cathodal electrophoretic mobility than the GPI-1b allele [181]. The presence of GPI-1BC is a demonstration of mosaicism of single myofibers. GPI-1BC appears as a hybrid band with intermediate electrophoretic mobility between its parental bands GPI-1BB and GPI-1CC.

The survival and development of donor cells in host muscles were demonstrated with agarose gel electrophoresis of the strain-specific isozymes of GPI at 6 months after MTT. Analyses of six test normal and eight test dystrophic solei showed that all contained both parental isozymes, but only half of each group exhibited GPI-1BC.

The presence of GP1-1CC in test dystrophic solei implied the survival and development of donor cells in host muscles. The normal myoblasts fused among themselves to form normal fibers that functioned within the dystrophic muscles. Furthermore, the presence of GPI-1BC in test solei substantiated intracellular mosaicism through fusion of host and donor cells. This initial evidence substantiates the mechanisms responsible for muscle improvement after MTT/HMGT (Figure 3). The demonstration of GPI-1CC and GPI-1BC, both of normal genotypic origin, in dystrophic host muscles provides the first evidence of genetic improvement. The latter is well-correlated with structural and functional improvement observed after MTT [145-148].

It is known that gene products encoded by local myonuclei are uniformly distributed throughout the myofiber syncytium [184]. Furthermore, heterokaryons containing nuclei from mouse muscle cells and human nonmuscle cells can be induced to produce proteins typical of human muscle [185]. Thus, in the MTT study it is likely that the normal donor myoblasts fused with host myofibers, sharing normal genes and restoring normal structure and function to the now mosaic myofibers. This latter contention, though partially supported by the presence of GPI-1BC, did require direct confirmation at the single cell level.

Whereas gel electrophoresis of muscle isozymes may be used to demonstrate genetic mosaicism of the myoblast-injected muscles, it does not allow correlation of genotypic constitution with phenotypic expression in single cells. The latter correlation requires the use of immunocytochemistry or nuclear labeling to localize, in mosaic fibers, donor myonuclei that contain the normal genome.

For immunocytochemical localization of host and donor nuclei within the injected muscles, polyclonal antibodies highly specific for GPI-1CC but not for GPI-1BB were produced [186-188]. These antibodies, when conjugated with nuclear stain and horseradish peroxidase (HRP), stained the nuclei of normal control muscles but not the dystrophic control muscles (Figure 4). Using this immunocytochemical procedure, Law et al. observed normal appearing mosaic fibers that contained host and donor nuclei 18 months after myoblast injection (Figure 4). Normal nuclei of donor origin were stained. Dystrophic nuclei of the host were not stained [147,148]. Whereas neighboring dystrophic fibers of the host were at different stages of degeneration, the mosaic fiber appeared histologically normal. The study provides strong direct evidence of gene therapy at the single cell level. Cell genetics of the dystrophic fiber is improved through incorporation of the normal nuclei with all of the normal genes. The dystrophic cell is replenished with normal copies of the defective gene. This genetic/structural correlation of the presence of donor nuclei of normal genotype in mosaic fibers of normal histology (Figure 4) provides the second evidence in support of the MTT/HMGT concept (Figure 3).

The mosaic muscles resulted from MTT also contained normal and dystrophic muscle fibers. The presence of genetically normal fibers demonstrates genetic improvement at the whole muscle level (Figure 6 C). This latter mechanism is better illustrated using gel electrophoresis showing the GPI-1CC band (Figure 6D).

Thus, with the use of isozymes of GPI as genotype markers for host and donor cells, both electrophoretography and immunocytochemistry indicated the survival and development of donor myoblasts in the host muscles. Donor myoblasts fused among themselves to form normal fibers. They also fused with host cells, sharing their normal gene pool to effect repairing in the genetically mosaic cell. These mechanisms have been explored as early as 1978 [50,96,145-148,183].

Analysis of sections of the mosaic fibers will allow the determination of how many genetically normal nuclei are necessary to convert the dystrophic muscle cell back to normal phenotype. In determining the minimal ratio of normal/dystrophic genotype mosaicism necessary to produce normal phenotype, we have developed, in addition to the antibodies specific for GPI-1CC [213-215], a vital dye muscle nuclear stain to label donor nuclei [189]. This method corroborates well with the GPI-1CC immunocytochemistry and is more reliable and convenient.

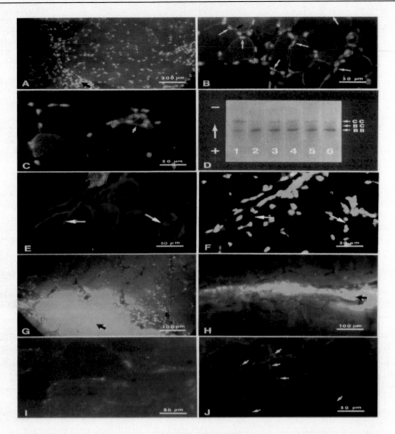

Figure 6. A. Fluorescent microscopy showing the wide and even distribution of F-G labeled donor myoblasts (yellow nuclei) in normal host muscle cross section. Arrow shows the site of injection. B. Host muscle showing mosaic muscle fibers as early as 7 days after myoblast injection. White arrows, donor nuclei; black arrows, host nuclei. C. Injected host muscle showing the fusion of donor myoblasts to form normal myotube (Arrow). D. All of the injected muscles show three different muscle fiber enzymes (GPI-1BB, BC, CC) in agarose gel electrophoresis. Lane 1, controls. E,F. Human myoblast transfer into mdx mouse muscle monitored by FG myoblast labeling, Hoechst 33342 nuclear counterstain, and dystrophin immunbocytochemistry. (F) Fluorescent microscopy showing the distribution of FG-labeled donor myoblast nuclei (yellow) and host nuclei (green) counterstained with Hoechst 33342. (E) Fluorescent microscopy of the same muscle section as (F), respectively, in which dystrophin (red) is observed with a Texas red filter. Arrows show fibers with distinct correlation between dystrophin immunocytochemistry and the presence of normal donor nuclei. G. (Control 1) Poor distribution as a result of poor injection technique. Arrow shows the site of injection. H.(Control 2) The distribution of FG-labeled dead myoblasts in the host muscle 7 days after injection. I. (Control 3) Host muscle injected with 0.01% F-G saline 7 days after injection. J. (Control 4) Auto fluorescence of host myonuclei. (Reproduced with permission from Fang et al.1991.)

The usage of GPI as genotype marker to follow the fate of donor myonuclei in host muscles is necessary for long-term studies, which in the case reported above, lasted up to 18 months after MTT [146-148]. However, the production of antibodies is extremely difficult and time consuming when the antibodies have to be specific enough to differentiate between isozymes [186-188]. For studies that involve shorter experimental periods, labeling the donor myonuclei with the vital dye Fluoro-Gold (FG) is more appropriate [189].

In vitro incubation with 0.01% FG (Fluorochrome Inc. Englewood, CO) for 16 h resulted in 100% nuclei labeling. Intensive fluorescence persisted following 9 days of subculture when labeled human myoblasts were injected into the quadriceps of mouse recipients immunosuppressed with cyclosporine A (CsA) [189].

FG was used as a donor cell marker to observe the status of donor cell nuclei in the host muscle. Donor myoblasts were found widely distributed in the injected host muscle. Myoblast fusion began one week after injection. Mosaic muscle fibers could be found in sections of muscles which had received myoblast injections. The incorporation of normal nuclei from cultured human myoblasts into host muscles of normal mice suggested that a similar procedure can be used to genetically improve dystrophic muscles. FG labeling was not observed in control muscles injected with an equal volume of FG-labeled dead myoblasts, 0.01% FG medium, or phosphate-buffered saline.

Aside from donor cell survival in an immunologically hostile host, cell fusion is the key to strengthening dystrophic muscles with MTT. To improve the fusion rate between host and donor cells, various injection methods aimed at wide dissemination of donor myoblasts were tested and compared. The goal was to achieve maximum cell fusion with the least number of injections.

The results indicate that delivery of myoblasts is best conducted by diagonal placement of needle into the host muscle with ejaculation of the myoblasts as the needle is withdrawn. This method of myoblast injection yields an even and wide distribution of donor myoblasts with a high rate of cell fusion. Myoblasts injected perpendicular to myofiber orientation are partially distributed. Myoblasts injected longitudinally through the core of the muscles and parallel to the myofibers are poorly distributed. Thus myoblast injection method regulates cell distribution and fusion [195].

Biochemical Improvement

To further examine the fate of the donor myoblasts and to further demonstrate genetic and biochemical improvement after MTT/HMGT, we developed a new technique which enables correlation of dystrophin expression with the location of donor versus host nuclei in the same sections of mdx mouse muscle injected with normal myoblasts.25 Myoblasts from C57BL/6J mice or from humans were labeled with 0.01% FG in Dulbecco's Modified Eagles Medium (DMEM) for 16 h at 37^{0}C before myoblast transfer. About 3 x 10^4 myoblasts were injected into the quadriceps muscles of mdx mice immunosuppressed with CsA. At 11, 21, or 25 days after myoblast transfer, injected muscles were dissected out and sectioned. These muscle sections were processed for dystrophin and then labeled with a fluorescent nucleus counterstain, 5 μg% Hoechst 33342 in phosphate-buffered saline (PBS), for 10 min at room temperature. FG labeling corresponding with Hoechst 33342 staining indicated survival of normal nuclei in dystrophic muscle. Dystrophin was found in the sarcolemma of myofibers containing FG-labeled nuclei but not of myofibers containing only Hoechst 33342 labeled nuclei (Figures 6E, F). Control muscle samples showed neither FG labeling nor dystrophin. The study demonstrates that the donor human and mouse myoblasts survived and developed in host mouse muscles after myoblast transfer, and that the localization of their normal nuclei correlates with dystrophin expression in muscle fibers of immunosuppressed mdx host mice. This genetic/biochemical correlation provides the third evidence in support of the MTT/HMGT concept (Figure 3), and confirms previous contention of genetic improvement as demonstrated using GPI gel electrophoresis and immunocytochemistry.

Structural Improvement

The first demonstration that cultured myoblasts can survive and develop in vivo in a dystrophic muscle after transplantation was reported by Law et al. in 1988 [145]. Genotypically normal (+/+) myoblasts were derived from limb bud explants of day 14 mouse embryos of the gpi-1c/c mice. The muscle primordia yielded samples consisting of 80% spindle-shaped myoblasts and 20% polygonal fibroblasts after proliferation in culture. Without purification, about 10^6 donor cells were injected into the right soleus of 20-day old normal or dystrophic mice.

Host and donors were histocompatible but exhibited different genotype markers. Donor cells produced GPI-1CC. Host cells produced GPI-1BB.

When compared with contralateral controls 6 months postoperatively, test dystrophic solei exhibited greater cross-sectional area and total fiber number (Figure 5). They contained more normal appearing and less abnormal-appearing fibers [145].

Improvement in histology correlated well with genetic improvement which was shown using GPI gel electrophoresis. Presence of GPI-1CC with or without hybrid isozyme GPI-1BC in these muscles implied the survival and development of donor myoblasts into normal myofibers, and fusion of normal myoblasts with dystrophic satellite cells to form genetically mosaic myofibers.

Injection of about 10^6 fibroblasts as a control for cell type resulted in less absolute number of fibers, higher percentage of abnormal fibers, and more connective tissues (Figure 5) in both test dystrophic and test normal solei [145]. This indicates that the structural improvement was indeed mediated through myoblasts and not through fibroblasts.

It should be noted that this study did not involve the use of CsA because of the histocompatibility between hosts and donors. This would indicate that the observed structural improvement was not caused by CsA.

Aside from the use of inbred mice that afford histocompatible MTT, the reality is that myoblasts exhibit MHC-1 surface antigens that provoke immunological rejection [190]. Furthermore, fully matched human donors and dystrophic recipients are rarely available [105,191]. Current technology would thus necessitate the inclusion of host immunosuppression to facilitate myoblast survival after transfer. Cyclosporine is the most widely documented immunosuppressant in transplantation studies [192]. FK 506 provides another alternative [193].

The first histoincompatible myoblast transfer into dystrophic muscles was reported in 1988 [146]. Donor myoblasts were clones of G8 cell line (ATCC) originally derived from limb muscles of the Swiss Webster mice. Host mice, either normal or dystrophic, belonged to the C57BL/6J-dy2Jdy2J strain. These mice were primed one week with CsA injected subcutaneously everyday at 50mg/kg body weight before receiving myoblasts. The same CsA treatment continued for 6 months after MTT. About 10^6 donor myoblasts were injected into each of the following muscle groups on both sides of the hosts: the quadriceps femoris, hamstrings, abductors, extensors, flexors, peroneal, and the external intercostal muscles. Control mice, both normal and dystrophic, received similar myoblast treatment but no CsA.

Histologically, there were no indications of the presence of donor cells in the myoblast injected normal muscles without CsA treatment. These muscle preparations, showing polygonal myofibers with peripheral nuclei and minimal intercellular connective tissue, were as normal as any intact normal controls. Similarly, the dystrophic muscles receiving myoblast injections but no CsA treatment did not differ from the intact dystrophic controls. However, both CsA-treated normal and dystrophic muscles showed immature and developing myogenic cells that were not observed in no-CsA-treated preparations and were thus likely to be donor in origin. Two months was not long enough for all of the donor cells to mature. Nonetheless, there was a significant improvement in muscle structure in the CsA-treated dystrophic mice as compared to the no-CsA-treated dystrophic ones, both receiving normal myoblasts. Dystrophic characteristics such as muscle fiber splitting, central nucleation, phagocytic necrosis, variation in fiber shape and size, and increase in intercellular connective tissues were rarely present in the CsA-treated dystrophic muscle receiving normal myoblasts. It should be noted that the action of CsA is one of an immunosuppressant, and that CsA does not improve muscle cell structure by itself [194]. The latter is especially obvious considering the positive results of histocompatible MTT with using CsA.

The survival and development of donor cells in host muscles were also demonstrated in another series of experiments in which only the right legs received myoblast injections, with the left legs serving as controls. The injected leg showed muscle enlargement which was not observable in the contralateral leg. Such muscle enlargement was present in the CsA-treated hosts but not in those without CsA treatment, regardless of whether the host was normal or dystrophic. These results were obtained from 12 mice from each of the four groups 2 months after myoblast injection [146].

Functional Improvement

Histocompatible Transfer

After 6 months, injection of 10^6 histocompatible cultured myoblasts into the 20-day-old dy2Jdy2J mouse soleus produced significantly greater muscle twitch tension, tetanus tension and wet weight than the contralateral unoperated control (Figure 7) [145]. Injection of fibroblasts instead of myoblasts caused significant reduction in twitch and tetanus tensions in the test dystrophic solei, although the test normal solei were unaffected. Results were obtained from 10 normal and 6 dystrophic mice.

The study demonstrated for the *first* time that cultured myoblasts could survive, develop in vivo, and function in a disease environment. It established a link between the cell culture and the in vivo systems. In vivo genetic complementation study on mammalian skeletal muscle had not been reported.

These results indicate that histocompatible MTT with cultured myoblast is safe and effective in improving mammalian dystrophic muscle function.

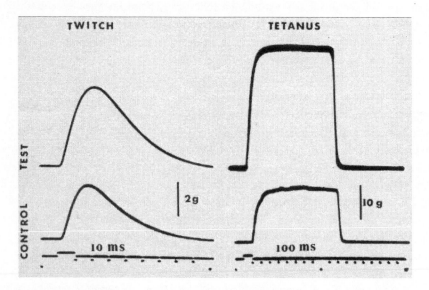

Figure 7. Mechnophysiology in vivo at 37°C showing significantly increased twitch and tetanus tensions for the myoblast-injected dystrophic soleus as compared to the contralateral uninjected dystrophic control.

Histoincompatible Transfer

The ideal situation was to develop healthy clone lines of normal myoblasts in reserve for injection. This was already available through the G8-1 cell line which was histoincompatible with the C57BL/6J hosts. G8-1 cloned myoblasts were purchased from ATCC. The initial injection study using these clones occasionally showed tumorigencity. Subsequently, we developed and used myoblast clones from Swiss Webster mouse embryos from which the original G8-1 clones were derived.

Immunosuppression was induced by daily subcutaneous injection of CsA at 50 mg/kg body weight. CsA was withdrawn after 6 months of treatment. The survival of cloned myoblasts in muscles of CsA-treated and non-treated C57BL/6J normal or dystrophic mice was examined.10-12 Donor myoblasts that produced GPI-1AA were injected multifocally via a 30 gauge needle into the major muscle groups of the calf in both legs: tibialis anterior and extensor digitorum longus representing the extensors, the triceps surae representing the flexors, the quadriceps, and the hamstrings. About 10^6 myoblasts were injected into each muscle group of the 20 to 30-day-old mice. The external intercostal muscles on both sides also received 10^6 normal myoblasts each as previously described. In vivo mechanophysiology with supramaximal nerve stimulation showed significant increase in tetanus tensions in myoblast injected dystrophic muscle groups of CsA-treated mice. The latter study included 12 normal and 19 dystrophic mice. The increase in tetanus tensions indicated that histoincompatible MTT is safe and effective in strengthening mammalian dystrophic muscles [146-148].

Behavioral Improvement

From 2 to 18 months after myoblast injection, eleven dystrophic mice showed such behavioral improvement that their locomotive patterns were indistinguishable from those of the unoperated normal mice [146-148]. Sporadic flexion associated with myotonia and flaccid extension of the hindlimbs was not seen. They were able to use their hindlimbs and toes. Their hindlimb muscles were strong enough to support them and to allow them to balance themselves on a glass rod and to climb out of a cage. Occasionally they would still walk on duck feet, but the mice could now run. Muscle bulk was increased in both legs and in the chest.

Five mice did not respond at all. Three other mice showed intermediate recovery 2 months after myoblast injection indicating that there was some functional improvement of the muscles. However, when they were tested on the glass rod, their hind-limbs were not strong enough to hold onto the glass rod. Sporadic flexion and flaccid extension of the hind-limbs could still be demonstrated.

One year after myoblast injection, the mice that showed significant behavioral improvement continued to be able to support themselves on their hind-limbs and walked normally. They could grasp the glass rod with their toes, and were able to balance themselves and moved along the glass rod.

The mice that showed intermediate improvement could now walk on the glass rod without showing sporadic flexion and flaccid extension of the hind-limbs. They continued to walk with duck feet.

Normal littermates treated similarly were hyperactive, showed enlarged intercostal and leg muscles, but were otherwise normal.

Before myoblast injection, four-month old dystrophic mice could not run the treadmill at 2 meters/minute. After myoblast injection, they could run at 2.8 meters/minute. The one that showed most improvement actually outran that speed and could jump out of the treadmill. Young dystrophic mice injected around one month of age could run at a speed of 7.1 meters/minute and could easily climb out of the treadmill, if the speed was slowed down to 2.8 meters/minute [146-148].

Life Prolongation

This study was remarkable in that because of the improvement of cell genetics, biochemistry, muscle function and animal behavior, the life span of the responding dystrophic mice (normally 8-9 months) was increased to nineteen months. This was likely due to strengthening of the intercostal and locomotive muscles, allowing the dystrophic mice to obtain enough oxygen, nutrients and exercise [202-204].

Among the five injected dystrophic mice that did not respond behaviorally, only one survived to a year after injection. Nevertheless, its life span was extended.

Perspectives

Two mechanisms (Figure 3) were responsible for these phenotype improvements. First, donor myoblasts fused among themselves, developed into normal fibers and replenished lost dystrophic myofibers. Second, normal myoblasts fused with dystrophic myogenic cells, sharing the normal genome to effect genetic repair at the cellular level.

These two mechanisms of genetic complementation were demonstrated using GPIs as genotype markers (Figure 6D). The presence of parental isozymes in the myoblast injected muscles indicated the survival and development of donor cells in host muscles. Furthermore, the presence of hybrid isozymes GPI-1BC indicated fusion between host and donor cells.

The immunocytochemical localization of host and donor nuclei within myofibers of the injected muscles using GPI polyclonal antibodies further substantiated the mechanism. These antibodies stained the nuclei of normal control muscles but not the dystrophic control muscles. Normal-appearing mosaic fibers containing host and donor nuclei could be observed eighteen months after myoblast injection (Figure 4). This genetic/structural correlation provides the second evidence in support of the MTT/HMGT concept. Analysis of sections of the mosaic fibers will allow the determination of how many genetically normal nuclei are necessary to convert the dystrophic muscle cell back to normal phenotype. The mosaic muscles also contained normal and dystrophic muscle fibers (Figure 5).

The third and final proof of concept utilizes genetic/biochemical correlation in which dystrophin induction was demonstrated in the sarcolemma of myofibers containing FG-labeled normal nuclei but not in myofibers containing only Hoechst 33342 labeled dystrophic nuclei (Figure 6).

Animal experimentation from 1975 to 1990 demonstrated that MTT/HMGT was safe and effective. The beneficial effect was not due to the use of CsA, fibroblasts or needle trauma. Normal myoblast injections provide long-term genetic complementation treatment for muscle degeneration in murine dystrophy. The procedure repairs degenerating cells and replenishes degenerated cells, thus normalizing cell genetics, biochemistry, structure, muscle function, animal behavior and life span.

Since the treatment design is based on development processes universal to all mammals, it has potential for clinical application to treat all types of muscle diseases. This animal experimentation lays the scientific groundwork for the development of a clinical treatment, with the promise of bringing restoration of function and quality of life to patients who suffer muscular dystrophy. Such treatment may potentially prevent or remedy muscle weaknesses in locomotive and respiratory muscles, thereby improving the quality of life and prolonging the life span of the patients.

Chapter II

MYOBLAST TRANSFER IN DMD SUBJECTS

SINGLE MUSCLE TREATMENT

Phase I MTT/HMGT clinical trial began on February 15, 1990, after lengthy reviews despite the initial protocol approval on April 7, 1989 [196]. *It was the first human gene therapy clinical trial* [197]. Cultured myoblasts were used as vehicles to deliver all of the normal genes into DMD myofibers to repair genetic defects. As a cell therapy, MTT/HMGT was to replenish the degenerated myofibers also.

The study, a single muscle treatment (SMT), was based on the safety and efficacy of MTT/HMGT previously demonstrated in the dydy, dy2Jdy2J and mdx mice. The randomized, double-blind study was designed to determine the survival, development and functioning of donor myoblasts in dystrophic muscles of DMD boys. We hypothesize that intramuscular injection of normal myoblasts can significantly improve the biochemistry, structure and function of dystrophic muscles. Our goal is to demonstrate the safety and efficacy of MTT/HMGT in humans.

The experimental design and the results of the SMT study had previously been published [98-101,198].

SUBJECTS AND METHODS

Approval

This study protocol received approval from 1) the Institutional Review Board of the University of Tennessee Memphis (UTM); 2) the Scientific Advisory and Administrative Committees of the Clinical Research Center in UTM; 3) the LeBonheur Children's Medical Center Institutional Review Board, and 4) the UTM Data and Safety Monitoring Board.

Subjects

Eleven 6 to 10-year-old boys previously diagnosed in different MDA clinics of having DMD on the basis of physical examination, muscle biopsy, serum CPK, electromyography and/or absence dystrophin were selected. They were in good general health and were not on any medication. They showed no evidence of renal or liver disease as judged by normal levels of BUN, creatinine, SGOT, SGPT and alkaline phosphatase.

Muscle Preparation

Before admission into the project, the DMD boys demonstrated at least 25% reduction in isometric twitch tension in their extensor digitorum brevis (EDB) muscles as compared to age-matched normal boys. The EDB was chosen because of its early involvement in dystrophy [199,200], its easy access for myoblast injection, and its distinct innervation as the last muscle innervated by the common peroneal nerve so that its mechanophysiological properties could be objectively measured in vivo without movement artifacts. Its small size necessitated fewer injections of myoblasts to effect improved muscle structure and function. Confined to a small muscle, donor cells could easily be located during biopsy three months after myoblast injection. Its relative insignificance protected the subjects from the loss of use of an important muscle, should adverse reaction occur which might necessitate the removal of the whole muscle. Its unique location on top of the foot protected the developing muscle fibers and neuromuscular junctions from undue stretches as a result of the contracture of the antagonistic muscles.

Donor Myoblasts

These were derived from cell culture of muscle biopsies from normal fathers, male guardians or brothers of the subjects. Female family members were not used as muscle donors since they might be carriers of DMD. All donors were previously screened for human immunodeficiency virus (HIV) and hepatitis B infection.

Under local anesthesia, about 1 g of muscle was surgically removed from the rectus femoris muscle of each donor using an open biopsy technique. The muscle biopsy was immediately dissociated with 0.1% collagenase (Sigma type II) and 0.2% crude trypsin (Sigma) in phosphate buffered saline, pH 7.3. The latter contained 5.4mM KCl; 144 mM NaCl; 5 mM Na phosphate; 25 mM glucose; 14 mM sucrose; 50 units/ml penicillin; 10 μg/ml streptomycin; and 1 μg/ml phenol red. Complete dissociation of 1 g of fresh skeletal muscle occurred in 45 minutes of stirring with three changes of the enzyme solution, alternated with three changes of neutralizing medium. The latter was composed of 100 parts of Dulbecco's Modified Eagle's Medium (DMEM-Gibco) containing 0.37% NaHCO3 and 4 mM glutamine, 10 parts horse serum (Gibco) and 1% antibiotic-antimycotic (Gibco).

Cells were then cultured in the neutralizing medium supplemented with 2 parts of chick embryo extract (Gibco). Myoblasts were fed with fresh medium every two days and were incubated in 7% CO_2.

Before myoblast transfer into human recipients, myoblasts were tested for their ability to migrate, align, fuse and form myotubes and immature myofibers that could contract spontaneously in vitro. Myotubes were immunocytochemically stained for myosin. Fusion medium consisted of 98% DMEM and 2% horse serum. In addition, about 106 myoblasts from each donor were injected into a leg muscle of a normal C57BL/6J mouse to determine if the myoblasts were tumorigenic. The mice were immunosuppressed with daily subcutaneous injections of Cyclosporine (Cy) (50 mg/kg body weight) and were killed four weeks after myoblast transfer. Injection sites were examined for tumors.

Myoblast Transfer

Myoblasts were rinsed in Dulbecco phosphate-buffered saline (DPBS) which was used as the carrier solution for myoblast injection and for sham injections. Injections of 10^6 cells each were delivered at eight foci into each test EDB. A total volume of 400 μl was injected. Four foci were injected per puncture of the skin.

Injection of an equal volume of DPBS into the control EDB was administered in a similar manner. Myoblast-injected EDBs were randomly selected by the injecting physician. All other participants in the study including the patients were unaware as to which side received the myoblasts.

Immunosuppression

All donors and recipients were HLA tested. Results from HLA testings were used retrospectively to evaluate the significance of histocompatibility differences in determining the likelihood of engraftment in this initial series of patients. Forty-eight hours prior to myoblast injection, patients began receiving Cy. Sandimmune® (Cy) was administered orally at 5 to 7 mg/kg [201,202] divided in two doses per day (Sandoz, 100 mg/cc dissolved in an olive oil-Labrafil base to be further diluted by milk, chocolate milk, or orange juice). The dosage was varied to reach a whole blood trough Cy level of 100 to 200 ng/ml, as measured by the fluorescence polarization method (Abbott TDX). Cy concentration initially was monitored weekly for 3 weeks and then monthly. Cy treatment continued for three months. Routine blood and urine tests were performed weekly and then monthly to evaluate renal and liver function. Tests included BUN, creatinine, SGOT, SGPT and blood pressure determinations.

Effect of Cy on Myoblasts

The goal of Cy therapy was to maintain a serum trough concentration of 100 to 200 ng/ml. [145,146] To determine if cell proliferation and fusion of donor myoblasts might be affected by such Cy concentration, a study was conducted to examine the cell count, protein content and the fusion rate of clone myoblasts when exposed to 0, 50, 100, 150, 200, 300 or 500 ng/ml of Cy in vitro. Myoblasts were cultured for twelve days. Cell counts and total protein contents were determined seven days after plating. The fusion rate was determined five days after changing to the fusion medium, and in the presence of 0, 200, 500 ng/ml of Cy only.

Functional Monitor

Three days prior to myoblast injection and three months after, the isometric twitch and maximum voluntary contraction of the left and right EDBs were measured. The twitch tensions were elicited through supramaximal stimulation of the peroneal nerve at the ankle, such that the extensor hallucis longus (EHL) could not be stimulated to contract. Even if the EHL contributed to the maximum voluntary contraction of the big toe, this contribution should cancel out when muscle contractions before and after myoblast transfer were compared. The maximum voluntary contraction yielded registers of tetani tensions. The tensions were measured in vivo with an Omega LCL-20 force transducer connected via a stiff wire looping around the big toe. Six readings of each measurement were taken and averaged. Movement artifact was minimized by securing the foot to a frame. The transduced electric signals were transmitted through a WPI Transbridge, a MacLab and displayed on an Apple Macintosh SE screen. Tension measurements were confirmed from signal traces copied with an Apple Macintosh Laser-writer Plus.

Structural Monitor

Muscle biopsies (5x3x3 mm3) were obtained by open biopsy method three months after myoblast injection. Sections were cut at 6 μm in a cryostat and stained with Modified Gomori Trichrome [145].

Biochemical Monitor

Dystrophin is a cytoskeletal protein absent in DMD muscle cell membrane. If donor myoblasts survive and develop in DMD host muscles, dystrophin immunocytochemistry can be used to monitor biochemical success as shown in mice [95,96].

The immunocytochemical staining for dystrophin followed the methods of Hoffman et al.15 and Bonilla et al.16 Muscle biopsies (30mm^3) of normal adults and of DMD boys were frozen in 2-methylbutane chilled in liquid nitrogen. Six-micron thick transverse sections were cut in a cryostat maintained at -20^0 C. Muscle sections were thawed on 0.5% gelatin-coated slides. They were then fixed for one minute at room temperature with acetone.

The sections were incubated for two hours with pre-centrifuged antidystrophin serum diluted 1:1,000 with 95% PBS and 5% horse serum. They were then washed three times in PBS. They were further incubated for 60 minutes in biotinylated donkey anti-sheep IgG (Amersham) diluted 1:100 with 95% PBS and 5% horse serum. After being washed three times in PBS, they were mounted with 50% glycerol in PBS and examined. Control sections were incubated with non-immune serum and were processed on the same slides in the same manner.

RESULTS

Myoblast Culture

After seven days in culture, the satellite cells released from the donor biopsy took on the spindle-shape characteristics of the myoblasts. Healthy myoblasts were selected for cloning. The myoblasts had the ability to migrate, align, undergo mitotic division and form myoblast clones. Myoblasts were harvested for injection between 20 to 30 days after culturing. When left alone in culture, the myoblasts fused together to form multinucleated myotubes. These myotubes possessed striations or sarcomeres. They contracted spontaneously and eventually pulled themselves away from the bottom of the culture flask. Immunocytochemical staining indicated that myotubes formed from fusion of these myoblasts contained the contractile protein myosin (Figure 2). Myoblasts injected into immunosuppressed mice survived and developed without any sign of tumorigenicity.

Due to Professor Law's move from the University of Tennessee Memphis to the Cell Therapy Research Foundation, complete data on muscle function, structure, and biochemistry were obtained from only 3 out of the 11 subjects that received SMT.

Functional Improvement

The EDB of 9-year-old DMD boys developed only about half of the amplitudes in twitch and tetanus tensions of the age-matched normal controls. Three months after myoblast injection, the myoblast-injected EDBs showed significant increases in tensions whereas sham-injected EDBs showed reductions. Functional improvement in maximum voluntary contraction ranged from 13%

with myoblasts derived from a ward (patient 1), to 30% (patient 2) and 80% (patient 3) from brothers [98-100,198].

Structural Improvement

Myoblast-injected EDBs showed gross anatomical improvement over the sham-injected EDBs. In the sham-injected muscle biopsies, dystrophic characteristics such as muscle fiber splitting, central nucleation, variation in fiber shape and size, infiltration of fat and connective tissue and phagocytic necrosis were significant. The myoblast-injected muscle biopsy contained larger fibers that were relatively uniform in fiber shape and size. There was very little intercellular connective tissue. Muscle fibers were polygonal in cross-section. Nuclei were peripherally located. Dystrophic characteristics, while present, were less apparent [98-100,198].

Biochemical Improvement

Both immunocytochemical staining and immunoblot revealed dystrophin in the myoblast-injected EDBs but not in the sham-injected EDBs. Dystrophin was immunocytochemically localized at the sarcolemma. This was not seen in the sham-injected muscle. Many muscle fibers with dystrophin in the myoblast-injected muscle showed normal appearances. They were polygonal in shape, and nuclei were peripherally located.

Clinical Tests

At no time during the 92 days after myoblast injection of the 11 subjects was there any sign of erythema, swelling or tenderness at the injection sites. Serial laboratory evaluation, including electrolytes, creatinine and urea, did not reveal any significant changes before or after MTT/HMGT. There was no clinical evidence of an adverse reaction to MTT/HMGT or to Cy.

DISCUSSION

This is the *first* study to have provided corroborative data on biochemical, structural and functional improvement of DMD muscles after MTT/HMGT. By virtue of its absence in DMD muscles, dystrophin can be used a biochemical marker to monitor MTT/HMGT success. The presence of dystrophin in myoblast-injected but not in the sham-injected muscles provided unequivocal evidence of the survival and development of donor myoblasts in the myoblast-injected muscles. Although correction of the primary genetic defect is demonstrated, such evidence cannot be extrapolated to indicate structural and functional improvement, which have to be demonstrated by themselves as in this study. MTT/HMGT is a safe and effective procedure to alleviate some of the biochemical, structural and functional deficits inherent in small muscles of DMD.

SMT began on February 15, 1990. It was the *first human gene therapy* clinical trial [98,197]. Cultured myoblasts were used to deliver all of the normal genes into DMD myofibers to repair genetic defects. Correction of the DMD genetic defect was published in July 1990, when dystrophin was found in the myoblast-injected DMD muscle [98]. Improvement in muscle structure and function after MTT/HMGT were also announced [205]. Two months later, Anderson announced the beginning of the single gene manipulation therapy. T cells from an ADA deficient SCID patient were transduced with the functional ADA gene and returned to the patient after expansion through culture [206,207]. Correction of ADA deficiency in the SCID patient [122,139] was published eight months after dystrophin replenishment was reported in myofibers of a DMD patient [197]. Anderson's success has sparked much hope for gene therapy.

Different HMGT techniques that accounted for success or failure, were employed in different laboratories. At the initiation of SMT, hardly any group besides Law's had published significant animal experimentation with MTT/HMGT. Like Karpati [208,209] in Montreal, Miller [102,210] in San Francisco used myoblasts cultured in commercialized laboratories away from the myoblast transfer suites. Donor myoblasts might have been subjected to changes of nutrients, temperature, pH, and sterility in transit. Myoblast purity was doubtful especially in the early studies. Karpati transferred 55 million cells with 55 injections into the biceps brachii. Miller transferred 100 million cells with 100 injections into the tibialis anterior. In both cases, cells were transferred at lower concentrations in which cells reportedly leaked from the sites of injection. In Law's later study, 312 million myoblasts were transferred through three injections into the tibialis anterior, at a concentration of 55.6×10^6 cells/mL.

Apart from fewer cells delivered at a lower concentration, the much larger numbers of injections spaced indiscriminately 1 cm apart undoubtedly introduced a higher risk of embolism and much more damage to the recipients' blood vessels, nerves, and muscles which were known to lack the normal ability to regenerate [211]. A traumatized nerve takes 6 to 8 weeks to regenerate. Myotubes formed from myoblast fusion within the first 4 weeks of MTT/HMGT required nerve innervation to survive. The trauma of injection could further mobilize macrophages to remove not only the degenerate but also the donor myoblasts. It is possible that repeated injections over several months would increase the possibility of triggering a general immune reaction to the donor cells and that they put the subject at greater risk. Such technique was used by Mendell in Columbus,Ohio.

LOWER BODY TREATMENT

With the SMT results partially confirmed [102,104,105,] the feasibility, safety, and efficacy of HMGT were assessed in an experimental lower body treatment (LBT) involving 32 DMD boys aged 6-14 yr, half of whom were nonambulatory [141,191]. The LBT protocol received approval from the Essex Institutional Review Board Inc in Lebanon, NJ, which is in compliance with the regulations of the Food and Drug Administration. The protocol was also approved by the Patient Participation Committee of the Baptist Memorial Hospital Medical Center in Memphis, TN.

Through 48 injections, five billion (55.6×10^6/ mL) normal myoblasts were injected into 22 major muscles in both lower limbs, in 10 minutes with the subject under general anesthesia. Ten subjects received myoblasts cultured from satellite cells derived from 1-g fresh muscle biopsies of normal males aged 9-21 yr. Donor myoblasts for the remaining 22 boys were subcultured from reserves frozen 1 mo to 1.5 yr ago.

Only four donors were known to have identical histocompatibility with their recipients. All subjects took oral doses of the immunosuppressant cyclosporine (Cy), beginning at 2 days before HMGT and lasting for 6 mo after HMGT to facilitate donor cell survival. There was no evidence of an adverse reaction to HMGT or Cy as determined by serial laboratory evaluations including electrolytes, creatinine, and urea.

Objective functional tests using the KinCom Robotic Dynamometer measured the maximum isometric contractile forces of the ankle plantar flexors (AF), knee flexors (KF), and knee extensors (KE) before HMGT and at 3, 6, and 9 mo after HMGT. The AF, being distal muscles and less degenerative than the KE and the KF, showed no decrease in mean contractile force 3 mo after HMGT, and progressive increases in force at 6 and 9 mo after HMGT.

At 9 mo after HMGT, 60% of the 60 AF examined showed a mean increase of 50% in force ; 28% showed no change; and only 12% showed a mean decrease in force of 29% when compared to the function of the same muscles before HMGT. The KF, being proximal muscles and more degenerative, showed no change in function at 9 mo after HMGT. The KE, being proximal and anti-gravitational, were most degenerative before HMGT. They showed no statistically significant change in force at 3 mo after HMGT but showed decreases at 6 and 9 mo after HMGT.

At 9 mo after HMGT, 23% of the 60 KE examined showed a mean increase of 65% in force; 22% showed no change; and 55% showed a mean decrease of 24% in force. When results of all muscle groups (AF, KF, KE) were pooled, there was no change in force at 3, 6, or 9 mo after HMGT versus before HMGT according to the Wilcoxon signed rank test.

The ambulatory subjects showed more muscle improvement than the non-ambulatory ones at various times after HMGT. Statistically significant progressive increase in force in the AF and arrest of weakening in the KF and KE were observed in the ambulatory subjects as early as 3 months and continued up to 9 months after HMGT.

The results indicate that 1) HMGT is safe; 2) HMGT improves muscle function in DMD: 88% of the AF, 49% of the KF, and 45% of the KE showed either increase in strength or didnot show continuous loss of strength 9 mo after HMGT; 3) LBT significantly strengthens the lower bodies in one-third of the 32 DMD boys, improving their locomotive ability and quality of life. The behavioral improvement subsided for insufficient dosage of myoblasts and continual upper body weakening. 4) the dosage used is more effective in the AF than in the KF, and is least effective in the KE; 5) more than 5 billion myoblasts are necessary to strengthen both lower limbs of a DMD boy between 6 to 14 yr of age; 6) the more degenerated proximal muscles will need more myoblasts per unit muscle volume than the distal muscles for HMGT to be effective; 7) HMGT is more effective in the younger, ambulatory subjects than in the older, nonambulatory subjects; 8) Cy is not responsible for the functional improvement, since muscle function continues to improve 9 mo after HMGT despite Cy withdrawal at 6 mo after HMGT; 9) Cy immunosuppression permits donor cell survival and development, without overt rejection symptoms, when properly managed; 10) myoblasts from frozen reserves are as effective as those from fresh muscle biopsies; 11) fifteen billion myoblasts can be cultured from a 1-g muscle biopsy; 12) billions of cultured myoblasts can be injected into subjects without tumor formation.

BETTER REPAIR THAN REPLENISH

Although donor myoblasts are known to fuse among themselves, forming normal myofibers to replenish degenerated ones, this mechanism is much less efficient than repairing degenerating myofibers through incorporation of donor myonuclei as a result of the fusion of host and donor cells [95,140,145,147,148,169,171]. Myonuclear counts of myotubes and teased myofibers suggest that between 200 to 500 myoblasts fuse to form a single myofiber. The myotube so formed has to be attached, vascularized, and innervated, with subsequent differentiation and development of cytoarchitecture before being functional. On the contrary, the host degenerating myofibers already have functioning blood, nerve and tendon connections and require about 20% normal nuclei within them to change the dystrophic characteristics to normal [147]. Accordingly, HMGT should be more effective in younger patients in whom dystrophy has not destroyed as many myofibers.

FROZEN OR FRESH

Donor myoblasts derived from frozen reserves are as effective as those from fresh muscle biopsies. The majority of the subjects (22 out of 32) received myoblasts from frozen reserves, and improvement was observed in this group as in the remaining 10 subjects. This finding substantiates the idea that cell lines of superior myoblasts can be established and stored in cell banks [146].23 Furthermore, myoblasts can be harvested from culture, frozen, and transported for use in HMGT clinics away from the cell banks.

CYCLOSPORINE

The use of Cy is necessary to provide initial suppression against rejection because myoblasts exhibit surface antigenic determinants. The latter are either masked or absent in myotubes and myofibers.29 The continuous increases in muscle function after Cy withdrawal in this study, and in the dy2Jdy2J mouse studies [146-148], indicate that it is not necessary to immunosuppress the HMGT recipient beyond 6 months, using half of Sandoz recommended Cy dosage (15 mg/kg/ body weight/day).

Cy is not responsible for the functional improvement because muscle function continued to improve in the AF and the KF despite Cy withdrawal. The progressive weakening of the KE further argues against the claim that Cy improves DMD muscle function. Other evidence indicating why Cy is not responsible for DMD functional improvement has already been reported [141].

DOSING OF CELLS

Judging from the results of this study, it will require at least 25 billion myoblasts to populate the major muscle groups of the whole body of a DMD boy for HMGT to show dramatic behavioral improvement and possible life-prolongation. Fewer myoblasts will be needed by the younger patients who demonstrate less degeneration and weakening. Perhaps the ideal age of HMGT treatment for DMD boys is between three to five years when muscle growth is rapid. The proximal muscles will require more myoblasts per unit volume muscle than the distal muscles for HMGT to be effective. Whereas many authors have questioned whether enough myoblasts can be cultured [94,96,127], it is obvious from this study that the demand can be met by taking two grams of donor muscle biopsy.

Indeed, HMGT is the first genetic treatment to have produced any functional improvement in humans, through incorporation of normal genes into genetically defective cells and through incorporation of genetically normal cells into the genetically abnormal organisms [101,141,191].

CONTROVERSIES

Gene therapy encompasses interventions that involve deliberate alteration of the genetic material of living cells to prevent or to treat diseases [246]. According to this FDA definition, the first MTT/HMGT on a DMD boy on February 15, 1990 marked the first clinical trial on human gene therapy [197]. In addition to fulfilling their primary muscle-building mission, the myoblasts served as the source and the transfer vehicles of normal genes to correct the gene defects of DMD.

A pioneering work [207,217,243] is often considered as the "first human gene therapy"; correction of the ADA deficiency study began on September 14, 1990 [207], two months after the MTT/HMGT correction of the DMD gene defect was published [256]. In the ADA protocol, T cells from a patient with a severe combined immunodeficiency disorder (SCID) were transduced with functional ADA genes ex vivo and returned to the patient after expansion through culture. In the MTT/HMGT protocol, primary culture of myoblasts derived from a muscle biopsy of a normal donor was injected into a muscle of the DMD subject to produce in vivo nuclear complementation. Both gene therapies utilize cell transplantation to treat diseases. The ADA protocol involved genetic modification and correction of the patients T cells with the adenosine deaminase gene whereas in the DMD protocol normal donor cells were used which were not genetically modified ex vivo.

Six years after the foremost MTT/HMGT, dystrophin was found in the myoblast-injected muscle but not in the sham-injected muscle (Figure 8) [262]. Six years is the longest period through which any gene therapy has sustained positive results. Despite cyclosporine withdrawal at 3 months after MTT/HMGT, myofibers expressing foreign dystrophin were not rejected. This is because dystrophin is located in the inner surface of the plasma membrane, and because mature myofibers do not exhibit MHC-1 surface antigens. Not only has the result demonstrated MTT/HMGT overall safety and efficacy in this single case, it also shows stability in the integration, regulation and expression of the dystrophin gene. The presence of dystrophin in the myoblast-injected but not in the sham-injected muscle provided unequivocal evidence of the survival and development of donor myoblasts in the myoblast-injected muscle.

In a randomized double-blind study involving three subjects, myoblast-injected EDBs showed increases in tensions whereas sham-injected EDBs showed reductions [101,257]. Both immunocytochemical staining and immunoblot revealed dystrophin in the myoblast-injected EDBs. Dystrophic characteristics such as fiber splitting, central nucleation, phagocytic necrosis, variation in fiber shape and size, and infiltration of fat and connective tissues were less frequently observed in these muscles. Sham-injected EDBs exhibited significant structural and functional degeneration and no dystrophin. Throughout the study, there was no sign of erythema, swelling or tenderness at the injection sites. Serial laboratory evaluation including electrolytes, creatinine, and urea did not reveal any significant changes before or after MTT/HMGT.

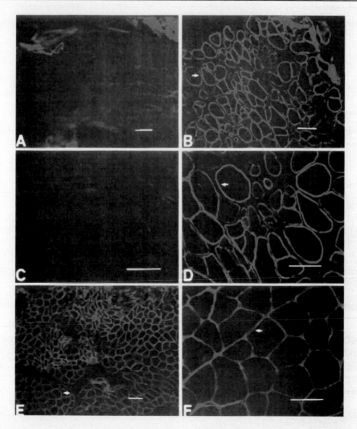

Figure 8. Immunocytochemical demonstration of dystrophin in DMD muscles 6 yr after MTT/HMGT. Dystrophin absent in sham- injected EDBmuscle (A, C), but present in the contralateral myoblaast- injected muscle (B, D). Dystrophin demonstrated at low (E) and high (F) magnification in normal control muscle. Arrows show dystrophin staining on sarcolemma. Cross-section; bar=100μm.

To reconcile these positive results with less convencing ones [102, 103, 105, 208, 210, 269, 271], several issues need to be addressed. To begin with, the use of large quantities of pure live myoblasts is a pre-requisite of successful MTT/HMGT. Except for Law's study [141,253], there is no published pictorial evidence to substantiate the purity, myogenicity and viability of the injected myoblasts as claimed.

Myoblast cultures are usually contaminated with fibroblast overgrowth. MTT/HMGT with such impure culture could lead to deposition of connective tissues rather than myofiber production. Culturing 50 billion pure human myoblasts for MTT/HMGT from two grams of muscle biopsy has only been reported by our team [261]. Other teams work at ranges of hundreds of millions of myoblasts.

In most studies [102, 103,105,208,210,269,271] myoblasts were transported frozen from the site of harvest, chilled for over two hours before being injected. Since myoblasts have a high metabolic rate, they could not have survived for two hours without significant nutrients, oxygen and proper pH, being closely packed in saline within a vial for transport. Determination of cell viability before HMGT were not conducted in these studies. Our myoblasts were injected into the subject within minutes of harvest, at the same location without transport.

HMGT studies that reported failure [102,103,105,208,210,269,271] subscribed to the fallacy of making 55 to 330 injections into a muscle the size of an egg, traumatizing indiscriminately the underlying nerves, muscle, and vasculature. These injection traumas boosted macrophage access and host immune responses [234]. They also induced fibrosis [221]. Surviving myoblasts fused within three weeks in small mouse muscles [95]. A nerve with multiple injuries could not regenerate soon enough through scar and connective tissues to innervate the newly-formed myotubes in a large human dystrophic muscle. Stabilization of muscle contractile properties in a similar situation is achieved by 60 days in the rat, and functional return is incomplete [219]. Non-innervated myotubes died within one week. Whatever few myotubes that developed in the unsuccessful MTT/HMGT studies could not compensate for the traumatized myofibers.

In the study yielding positive results, 5 to 8 x 10^8 pure myoblasts were delivered with eight injections into the biceps brachii without nerve injury [258,261]. Contrarily, in another study, 55 sites, each 5 mm apart, distributed in 11 rows and 5 columns, were injected throughout the depth of each biceps of 5- to 9- year old boys [369]. This was repeated monthly for six months. Axonal sprouts, myotubes and neuromuscular junctions that take six weeks to mature [233] were repeatedly traumatized by a total of 330 injections until the biceps, with or without myoblast/cyclosporine, were irreversibly damaged or destroyed. The result: no functional difference between myoblast- and sham-injected muscles [269].

Once injected, the myoblasts are subjected to scavenger hunt by macrophages for up to three weeks. This is because myoblasts exhibit MHC-1 surface antigens [190,232] that become absent after cell fusion. The latter occurs between one to three weeks after myoblast injection [95]. An allowance in the number of injected myoblasts has to be made to satisfy the unavoidable scavenger process. As reflected in the small numbers of myoblasts injected in unsuccessful studies, it appears that either such allowance was not considered or that the teams were not able to produce larger quantities of pure myoblasts. Although myoblast loss can be minimized by down-regulating macrophage activity [235], such additional compromisation of the host immune system may lead to higher risk of infection, since MTT/HMGT subjects are already taking immunosuppressants.

The less successful MTT/HMGT teams focused on immunosuppression to prevent T-lymphocyte proliferation and antibody production without overcoming the primary hurdle of providing enough pure and live myoblasts. A basic study indicates that cyclophosphamide did not permit myoblast engraftment in the mouse [290], and a MTT/HMGT clinical trial was conducted without success using cyclophosphamide immunosuppression [208]. Cyclosporine [256] and potentially FK506 [247] remain the immunosuppressants of choice for MTT/HMGT. Results could have been more positive if either was employed in the study of Tremblay et al. [103,105].

All of these single muscle MTT/HMGT studies had begun before the FDA established policies and regulations for cell/gene therapies. Our studies are the only ones that received permission for an investigational new drug application approval on MTT/HMGT for treatment of multiple muscles. As a cell/gene therapy, all American MTT/HMGT clinical trials must come under FDA purview.

WHOLE BODY TREATMENT

Dose Escalation

Beginning with 8 million myoblasts into a small foot muscle, our team proceeded to test 5 billion cells into 22 leg muscles, 25 billion cells into 64 body muscles, and now 50 billion cells into 82 muscles. With over 280 procedures having been conducted to date, the complete safety of the MTT/HMGT procedure has been proven. There have been no adverse reactions or side effects.

Myoblasts	Muscles	Subjects
8 million	1	11
5 billion	22	32
25 billion	64	40
50 billion	82	197

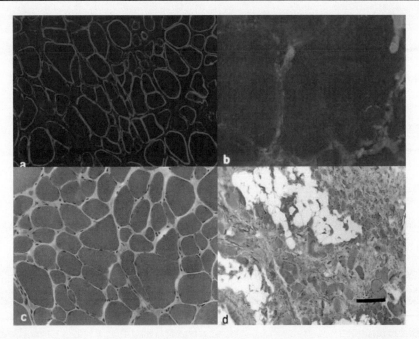

Figure 9. At 9 mo after HMGT, dystrophin was found in the myoblast- injected muscle (a) with histological improvement (c), but not in the placebo-injected muscle (b), which showed fat, connective tissues and minimal amount of myofibers (d).

The 25 Billion Myoblast Protocol

Under FDA purview, MTT/HMGT Phase II clinical trials began on DMD. The whole body trial (WBT) consisted of injecting 25 billion myoblasts in two MTT/HMGT procedures separated by 3 to 9 mo. Each procedure delivered up to 200 injections or 12.5 billion myoblasts to either 28 muscles in the upper body (UBT) or to 36 muscles in the lower body (LBT). A randomized double-blind portion of the study was conducted on the biceps brachii or quadriceps. Subjects took oral cyclosporine for 3 months after each MTT. One infantile facioscapulohumeral dystrophy and 40 DMD boys aged 6 to 16 received WBT in the past 36 months with no adverse reaction.

Nine months after MTT/HMGT immunocytochemical evidence of dystrophin were demonstrated in 18 of the 20 DMD subjects biopsied (Figure 9). Dystrophin positive sections showed less dystrophic characteristics than dystrophin-negative ones (Figure 9). Forced vital capacity increased by 33.3% and maximum voluntary ventilation increased by 28% at 12 months after UBT [261].

Plantar flexion showed an increase of 45% in maximum isometric contraction force in 12 months in the DMD subjects when compared to the natural deterioration. Behavioral improvements in running, balancing, climbing stairs and playing ball were noted [259-261,263,264]. Notable was a 16-yr-old DMD subject who continued to walk without assistance and capable of driving an automobile by himself.

The 50 Billion Myoblast Protocol

This study involves a one time injection of 50 billion myoblasts into 82 muscles with 179 skin punctures, approved by the FDA for subjects with DMD, Becker MD and Limb-girdle MD [339]. Over 190 subjects who underwent this protocol have experienced no adverse reaction. For the DMD subjects aged 5 to 16, there was a significant increase in the maximum isometric force generated by the plantar flexor muscles at 3, 6, and 9 months after HMGT.

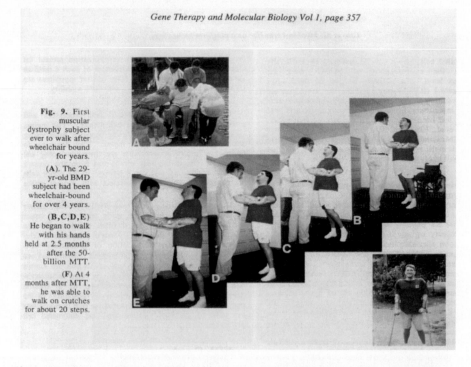

Gene Therapy and Molecular Biology Vol 1, page 357

Fig. 9. First muscular dystrophy subject ever to walk after wheelchair bound for years.

(A). The 29-yr-old BMD subject had been wheelchair-bound for over 4 years.

(B,C,D,E) He began to walk with his hands held at 2.5 months after the 50-billion MTT.

(F) At 4 months after MTT, he was able to walk on crutches for about 20 steps.

Figure 10. First muscular dystrophy subject ever to walk on crutches after wheelchair bound for 4 years.

This functional improvement is more pronounced with the 50-billion HMGT than with the 25-billion HMGT, indicating that it is dose-dependent. Thus, in the 25-billion HMGT, 800 million myoblasts were injected into the plantar flexors, producing a mean 61% increase in force at 15-months after MTT/HMGT. With the 50 billion HMGT, 50% more myoblasts were injected, projecting a 10% greater increase in force at 15 months after HMGT.

Elevated serum creatine kinase (CK) has traditionally been used to diagnose muscle degeneration, notable in DMD [300]. The initial 22 DMD subjects, mean ages 10.7-yr-old and, median age 9.9 yr-old, showed a 19.3% increase in serum CK within 3 months before HMGT. This trend was reversed after HMGT, and the serum CK declined at a steady rate of 48.7% over 12 months. This result provides strong evidence that HMGT repairs muscle cell membrane leakage of enzymes. This contention is further substantiated by similar findings with another muscle enzyme AST, aspartate aminotransferase.

The breakthrough came when a 29-yr-old Becker MD (BMD) subject began to walk, with his hands being held, beginning at 2.5 months after the 50-billion HMGT. He had previously been diagnosed repeatedly with BMD. He had been non-ambulatory and required the use of a wheelchair for over four years as documented in his medical record. He began walking with assistance a total of eight steps at 3 months after HMGT. This ability increased with time, reaching 60 steps at eight months after HMGT. He began to stand and walk with his crutches at four months after HMGT (Figure 10). Eventually he married, had a daughter and has led a quality life.

Chapter III

HUMAN MYOBLAST GENOME THERAPY AND THE REGENERATIVE HEART

Heart muscle degeneration is the leading cause of debilitation and death in humans. It is the common pathway underlying congenital and infectious cardiomyopathies, myocardial infarction, congestive heart failure, angina, coronary artery disease and peripheral vascular disease, all of which constitute the cardiovascular diseases. Global healthcare spending on the latter topped $280 billion in 2001. In the United States alone, approximately $186 billion is spent every year in treating some 60 million cardiovascular disease patients. About 50% of the 5 million plus patients suffering congestive heart failure will die within 5 years of diagnosis.

Bioengineering the regenerative heart may provide a novel treatment for cardiovascular diseases. Through endomyocardial injections of cultured skeletal myoblasts, the latter spontaneously transfer their nuclei into cardiomyocytes to impart myogenic regeneration. Injected myoblasts trans-differentiate to become cardiomyocytes. Donor myoblasts also fuse among themselves to form new myofibers, depositing contractile filaments to improve heart contractility. These myofibers contain satellite cells with regenerative vigor to combat heart muscle degeneration. The proof of concept is described below.

Human myoblasts transduced with $VEGF_{165}$ and Angiopoietin-1 genes produced six times more capillaries in porcine myocardium than placebo. Xenograft rejection was not observed for up to 30 weeks despite cyclosporine discontinuation at 6 weeks. Cyclosporine usage may be changed to 2 weeks in view of new findings. First in Man (FIM) studies using cGMP-produced pure myoblasts of autogenic and allogenic origins are documented. Pros and cons of autografts vs. allografts are compared to guide future development of Heart Cell Therapy using HMGT.

HEART MUSCLE REGENERATION

Heart muscle degeneration cascades with cardiomyocyte membrane leakage, uncontrolled Ca 2+ influx, mitochondrial ATP shutdown, inability to exude Ca 2+ through the cell surface and to reabsorb Ca 2+ into the sarcoplasmic reticulum, myofibrillar hypercontracture and disarrangement. Apoptosis ensues. Fibroblasts proliferate and infiltrate. The heart muscle, which was once populated by live cardiomyocytes with proteinaceous contractile filaments such as myosin, actin, troponin, tropomyosin, is now partially occupied by fibrous scars that are incapable of electric conduction, mechanical contraction and revascularization. These scars continue to exert a negative compliance on the heart, and the circulation, despite remodeling occurs after a myocardial infarction.

NATURAL HEART MUSCLE REPAIR

Ultimately heart muscle degeneration results in loss of live cardiomyocytes, contractile filaments, contractility, heart function and healthy circulation. The damaged heart responds by cell division of cardiomyocytes. However such regenerative capacity is hardly significant. Cardiomyocytes in culturo will undergo no more than three to five divisions, yielding an insufficient number of cells to repopulate any myocardial infarct.

Cardiomyocytes do not multiply significantly because the human telomeric DNA repeats [294] in these terminally differentiated cells are minimal. Telomerasing cardiomyocytes in vivo still remains a technical challenge. Without significant mitotic activity, surviving cardiomyocytes cannot provide enough new cells to deposit the contractile filaments necessary to maintain normal heart function.

The degenerative heart also transmits biochemical signals to recruit stem cells from the stroma and the bone marrow in an attempt to repair the muscle damage. This process can be augmented with stem cell transplants. Being pluripotent, embryonic or adult stem cells exhibit uncontrolled differentiation into various lineages to produce bone, cartilage, fat, connective tissue, skeletal and heart muscles (Figure 1). Because fibroblast growth factor level is elevated in the degenerative heart, much of the recruited stem cells differentiate to become fibroblasts instead of cardiomyocytes, thus depositing fibrous scars and not contractile filaments of muscles.

Despite the claimed success of transmyocardial revascularization using laser, angiogenic factors and genes, the damaged myocardium really needs additional live myogenic cells to deposit contractile filaments to regain heart function, preferably before fibroblast infiltration, which leads to scar formation.

MYOCARDIAL CELL TRANSPLANTATION

Myocardial cell transplantation is intended to compensate for the loss of cardiomyocyte number and aims to limit and/or reverse the consequences of contractile dysfunction of a damaged left ventricle [295-298]. These effects could be related directly to the injected cells or mediated indirectly by angiogenic or growth factors secreted by transplant cells [299-301]. More recently, transplantation of cells with inherent ability to secrete growth factors or genetically modulated cells carrying angiogenic growth factors is being assessed with the added consequence of angiogenesis concomitant with myogenesis [302-307]. The techniques for cardiac regeneration appear promising and offer alternative methods for the treatment of ischemic heart disease [308,353].

CHOISE OF CELL

Studies in cellular cardiomyoplasty have used embryonic stem cells, adult and fetal cardiomyocytes, fibroblasts, smooth muscle cells, mesenchymal stem cells, and myoblasts [309-316]. Adult and fetal cardiomyocyte implants produced viable and stable grafts in small mammals [317]. They form intercalated discs and gap junctions after grafting, suggesting electromechanical coupling of these cells with the host myocardium [318]. However, the use of embryonic stem cells and fetal cardiomyocytes in humans raises ethical and availability issues.

Myoblast Suitability

The advantages of using autologous skeletal myoblasts are availability, the lack of immunologic barriers to the transplantation process, which precludes the need for immunosuppression to allow donor cell acceptance by the host. Myoblasts can be genetically modified in vitro to deliver angiogenic cytokines and growth factors to encourage angiomyogenesis.

Animal studies have shown that grafted myoblasts form myotubes in the myocardium and eventually mature to become myofibers with contractile apparatus. These results have been confirmed in humans [319,320]. The regenerates acquire a fatigue-resistant slow-twitch muscle phenotype which is more suited to perform the cardiac work load. Transplantation of myoblasts produces significant functional improvement in damaged hearts [295,298,321-323]. There have been contradicting reports on the differentiation of myoblasts into cardiomyocyte-like cells with intercalated discs [324]. It is doubtful if the injected myoblasts make any meaningful electromechanical connections with host cardiomyocytes through gap junctions [325].

World's *First* Human Myoblast Transfer into the Heart

Being terminally differentiated, cardiomyocytes do not divide significantly to regenerate the myocardium. Stem cells transplant posts ethical issues of abortion and technical uncertainties as to whether these pluripotent cells will absolutely differentiate into cardiomyocytes and not osteoblasts, chondrocytes or others. We present the first successful endovascular transfer of human myoblasts into the porcine myocardium. Porcine hearts highly resemble those of humans and are more prompt to fibrillate upon minor injury.

Following International Animal Care guidelines, a 100-lb juvenile female pig was anesthetized. Access was obtained via the right femoral artery using cutdown technique. Catheter advance into the left ventricle through the aorta was guided with fluoroscopy followed by endomyocardial mapping with the electromagnetic NOGA system (Biosense Webster Inc, Johnson & Johnson).

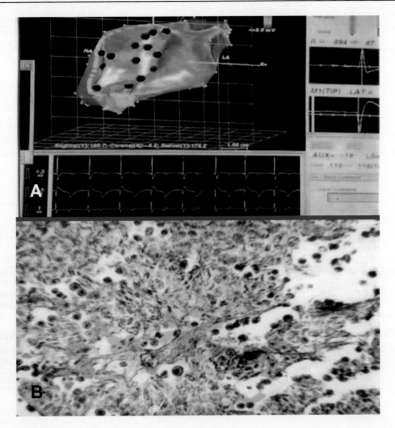

Figure 11. World's first human myoblast injections into the porcine heart to determine feasibility/safety and injection parameters for the MyoStar catheter and the process of heart cell therapy.

Approximately 10^9 human myoblasts were injected through a needle timed to protrude 6 mm from the tip of the catheter into the myocardium. Twenty injections were made at different locations within 40 minutes, having volumes of 0, 1, 0.2, 0.3, 0.5, 1.0 ml, and cell concentration of $100X10^6$/mL (Figure 11A). Heart rate, electrocardiogram and temperature were continuously monitored. Other than transient short runs of ventricular ectopy, the pig remained in stable condition throughout the injection period. There was no significant change in the parameters monitored. Vital dye staining of the myoblasts before versus after the procedure showed no significant difference in cell viability. Furthermore, cell passage through the injection catheter showed less than 5% of cell death.

At the completion of the procedure, the pig was sacrificed and the heart processed for histological examination. Transmyocardial perforation was not observed. Numerous prominent round and mononucleated human myoblasts were found widely and evenly distributed throughout the apex and the lateral wall of the pig left ventricle where the myoblasts were injected (Figure 11B). This study provides the first direct evidence demonstrating the feasibility and safety of endovascular delivery of human myoblasts into the porcine heart using the NOGA catheter injection system.

This *first* human myoblast transfer into the heart revealed that it was safe to administer one billion myoblasts at 100×10^6/ml through the Myostar catheter of the NOGA system (Biosense Webster Inc) using 20 injections at different locations inside the left ventricle of a swine [438]. It was determined that 0.3 ml to 0.5 ml would be the optimal volume per injection. EKG was normal throughout the study without arrhythmia.

THE REGENERATIVE HEART

The goal to bioengineer the regenerative heart seems to be within reach with HMGT. Five grams of muscle biopsies would be taken from both quadriceps of a heart patient with age ranging from 40 to 90, culturing approximately one billion myoblasts in four weeks and then injecting or surgically implanting these cells just inside the non-vascularized infracted myocardium.

Heart Cell Therapy (HCT) [328], as this is called, is administered with the vision that the myoblasts will survive, develop and function as aliens in the heart, and their nuclei as aliens within cardiomyocytes and myofibers. The myocardial aliens are newly formed skeletal myofibers that contribute to cardiac output through production of contractile filaments. They are donor in origin and as skeletal myofibers will have satellite cells and regenerative capability. The cardiomyocyte aliens are donor myoblast nuclei carrying chromosomes with long telomeric DNA subunits that are essential for mitosis. Upon injury of the trans-differentiated or heterokaryotic cardiomyocyte, the myoblast regenerative genome will be activated to produce foreign contractile filaments such as myosin and actin.

PROOF OF CONCEPT

Human myoblasts were manufactured according to our inhouse SOP's and trade secrets with a license of the U.S. Patent No. 5,130,14110 and with a license of the Singapore Patent No. 3449011 (WO 96/18303). This method of culture yielded purity of 99% by human desmin immunostaining (Figure 12). From 2g of human muscle biopsy, 50 billion pure myoblasts are produced routinely in our GMP facilities in about 45 days (Figure 13).

In the myogenesis study, cultured myoblasts derived from satellite cells of human rectus femoris biopsies were transduced with retroviral vector carrying Lac-Z reporter gene, and about 75% of the myonuclei were successfully transduced. Trypan blue stain revealed >95% cell viability immediately before injection.

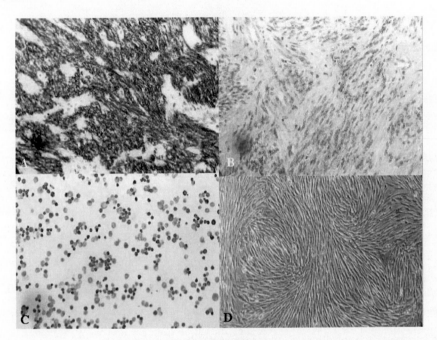

Figure 12. Human desmin immunostain for myoblast purity. (a) Positive control of leiomyosarcoma, staining brown. (b) Negative control. (c) Pure human myoblasts immunostained with desmin. (d) Pure human myoblasts in culture.

A porcine heart model of chronic ischemia was produced by clamping an ameroid ring around the left circumflex artery. Four weeks later, the heart was exposed by left thoracotomy. Twenty injections (0.25ml each) containing 300 million myoblasts, or 5ml total volume of basal DMEM as control, were injected into the left ventricle intramyocardially. Left ventricular function was assessed using MIBI-Tc99m SPECT scanning one week before injection to confirm myocardial infarction, and at 6 weeks after injection.

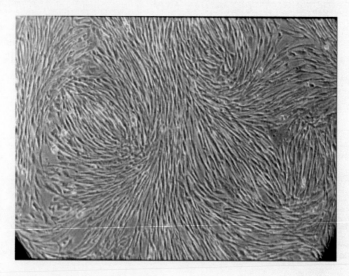

Figure 13. Pure myoblasts for MTT/HMGT.

Animals were maintained on cyclosporine at 5 mg/kg body weight from 5 days before, until 6 weeks after cell transplantation. The animals were euthanized at 6 weeks to 7 months post-operatively, and the hearts were processed for histological, immunocytochemical and ultrastructural studies.

Histological examination of myoblast-injected myocardium showed cardiomyocytes containing Lac-Z positive nuclei (of donor origin) after 12 weeks (Figure 14B). More than 80% of the Lac-Z positive cardiomyocytes immunostained positively for human myosin heavy chain (Figure 14A). The human genome was integrated (Lac-Z labelled nuclei) and expressed (myosin immunostain) in the porcine myocardium.

Donor myoblasts trans-differentiated to become cardiomyocytes that are characterized by having four to five nuclei each. The control heart without myoblast injection did not show Lac-Z positive myonuclei nor human myosin (Figure 14C). Triple stain of myoblast-injected myocardia demonstrated multinucleated heterokaryons containing human and porcine nuclei with expression of human myosin (Figure 15). Electron microscopy demonstrated human myotubes and skeletal myofibers with satellite cells in the porcine myocardium (Figure 16).

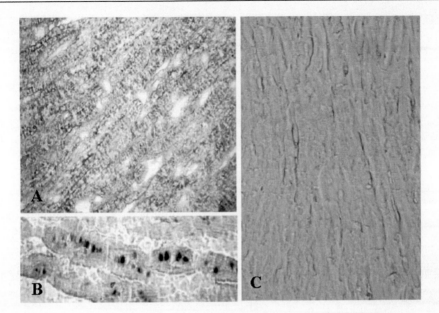

Figure 14. (a) Brownish immunostain of human myosin in porcine myocardium 12 weeks after human myoblast injection. (b) Cardiomyocytes each with 4 to 6 LacZ-positive nuclei and human myosin stain, indicative of their being donor or myoblastic in origin. (c) Negative immunostain (gray) of human myosin in porcine myocardium sham-injected without myoblasts.

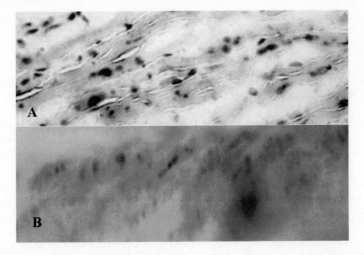

Figure 15. (a) Heterokaryons derived from fusion of porcine cardiomyocytes and human myoblasts showing LacZ-positive human myoblast nuclei (bluish green) and porcine cardiomyocyte nuclei (purple) in the heterokaryotic synytium. (b) These heterokaryons expressed human myosin heavy chain.

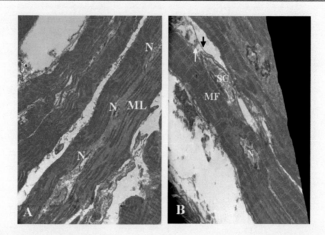

Figure 16. Electron microscopy of the myoblast-injected porcine myocardium showing (a) myotubes with central nuclei and myfibril (ML) deposits, and (b) skeletal myofiber with satellite cell (SC) and nucleus (N). The satellite cell is located between the basement membrane (black arrow) and the plasma membrane (white arrow). Sarcomeres show proper alignment of newly formed contractile filaments.

3 Mechanisms of Heart Cell Therapy/ Proof of Concept
Xenografts of Lac-Z labelled __human__ myoblasts into 50 __porcine__ hearts

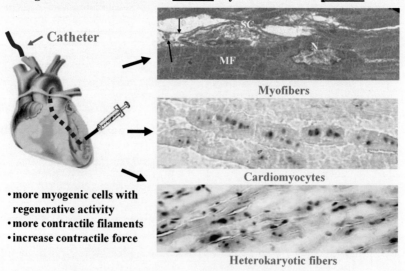

Figure 17. Proof of concept for HMGT to treat heart muscle degeneration, showing the fate of implanted human myoblasts into porcine myocardia. Three mechanisms were identified.

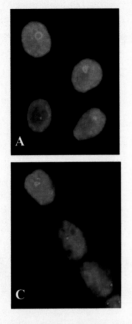

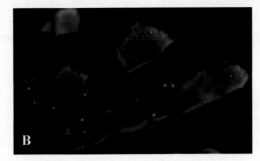

A. **Human Myoblasts. FISH probes specific for human chromosomes 22.**
B. **Control pig myocardium with no myoblast implant. FISH probes for human chromosomes 22 and for pig chromosomes 1 and 10.**
C. **Pig myocardium with myoblast implants showing heterokaryotic cardiomyocyte.**

Figure 18. FISH probes to demonstrate heterokaryotic cardiomyocyte.

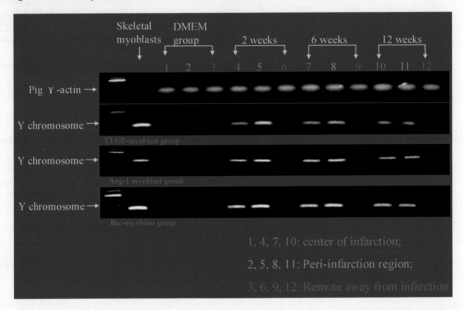

Figure 19. PCR analysis for detection of human Y chromosome in female pig heart. 1, 4, 7, 10: center of infarction; 2, 5, 8, 11: Peri-infarction region; 3, 6, 9, 12: Remote away from infarction.

Three myogenesis mechanisms were elucidated as proof of concept with 50 human/porcine xenografts using cyclosporine as immunosuppressant. Some myoblasts trans-differentiated to become cardiomyocytes. Others transferred their nuclei into host cardiomyocytes through natural cell fusion. As yet others formed skeletal myofibers with satellite cells. De novo production of contractile filaments augmented heart contractility (Figure 17) [351,352].

Laser nuclear capture together with single nucleus RT-PCR was performed to delineate host and donor nuclei. In situ hybridization using fluorescent DNA probes specific for human Y-chromosome and chromosomes 1&10 for pig were used to demonstrate nuclear mosaicism (Figure 18). The implantation of human myoblasts derived from young males into female pigs provides additional demonstration of donor cell survival and development in the host muscles (Figure 19).

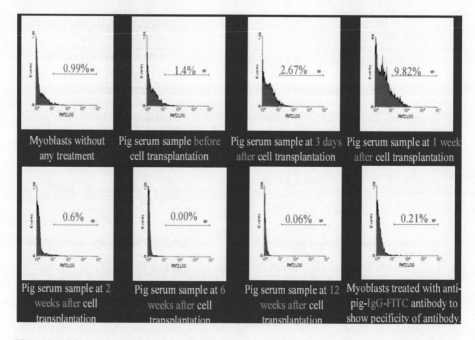

Figure 20. Pig immuno-tolerance with human myoblasts -transient presence of pig anti-human skeletal myoblast antibody. A. Myoblasts without any treatment. B. Pig serum sample before cell transplantation. C. Pig serum sample at 3 days after cell transplantation. D. Pig serum sample at 1 week after cell transplantation. E. Pig serum sample at 2 weeks after cell transplantation. F. Pig serum sample at 6 weeks after cell transplantation. G. Pig serum sample at 12 weeks after cell transplantation. H. Myoblasts treated with anti-pig-IgG-FITC antibody to show specificity of antibody.

Discontinuation of cyclosporine after 6 weeks prompted no xenograft rejection for up to 30 weeks. There was a transient elevation of the porcine anti-human- myoblast antibodies at one week after the xenograft (Figure 20). The antibody level subsided at the second week after HMGT, indicating that no more than two weeks of cyclosporine mmunosuppression would be necessary for human/pig xenografts. Modification of the cyclosporine administration protocol will be implemented accordingly in the future.

THERAPEUTIC ANGIOGENESIS

Therapeutic angiogenesis improves tissue ischemia by supplementing and supporting the intrinsic process of angiogenesis [354]. Besides direct administration of angiogenic growth factor proteins, injection of naked DNA, non-viral vectors and viral vector constructs carrying angiogenic genes have been used. A novel approach is to achieve therapeutic angiogenesis through cell mediated gene transfer. Genetically modulated cells carrying exogenous genes encoding for angiogenic factors and the cells with inherent ability to secrete angiogenic cytokines, such as bone marrow stem cells, embryonic stem cells and endothelial progenitor cells, have been used to achieve revascularization.

This review discusses proof of the concept pre-clinical studies and phase-I /II human trials using $VEGF_{165}$, and cellular angiogenesis at length in the light of the literature and analyzes the problems and considerations of these approaches as a treatment strategy in the clinical perspective for the treatment of ischemic heart disease.

Angiogenesis and vasculogenesis are primarily responsible for the development of the vascular system in the embryo. Whereas vasculogenesis involves angioblasts for the in situ new vessel development, angiogenesis occurs by sprouting of the already present primitive vasculature using previously differentiated cells [331]. A third mechanism that contributes to the development of collateral vessels is arteriogenesis through remodeling of the existing arterioles [329]. Angiogenesis is an integral part of many of the physiological and pathological processes, and angiogenesis is controlled by various factors that induce or inhibit blood vessel formation. Disruption of the natural balance between the pro- and anti-angiogenic factors results in pathological angiogenesis with abnormal blood vessel formation.

Therapeutic angiogenesis exploits the natural process for enhanced neovascularization [333]. Apart from direct administration of angiogenic proteins, naked plasmid and viral vector constructs carrying angiogenic genes have been used. Recent studies have suggested therapeutic angiogenesis through cell-mediated gene transfer and by stem cell transplantation. The transplantation of genetically modified cells serves as a reservoir to produce biologically active angiogenic factors in a localized and sustained pattern. Similarly, the application of stem cells not only can derive new vessel formation, but also differentiate into cardiomyocytes to restore injured myocardium.

This review summarizes the recent progress in therapeutic angiogenesis in conjunction with myogenesis, and critically analyzes the problems and considerations of this approach as a treatment strategy in the clinical setup for the treatment of myocardial infarction.

VEGF$_{165}$PROTEIN DELIVERY

The imbalance between supply and demand for oxygen in the hypoperfused myocardium up-regulates the expression of pro-angiogenic factors and their receptors [334,335]. VEGF$_{165}$ is the major angiogenic factor involved in physiological as well as pathological angiogenesis [330]. The neovascularization is mainly achieved by endothelial cell proliferation triggered through VEGF$_{165}$ receptors, especially the VEGF$_{165}$ receptor-2 [337]. VEGF$_{165}$ induces nitric oxide production and cGMP accumulation in cultured endothelial cells through the activation of endothelial nitric oxide synthetase (eNOS) [338]. The important functions of these two mediators are vasodilatation, inhibition of smooth muscle proliferation, anti-platelet accumulation and inhibition of leukocyte adhesion, leading to vascular protection [336]. Some of the factors stimulate angiogenesis through the induction of VEGF$_{165}$.

We have studied the potential of human myoblasts carrying human VEGF$_{165}$ for myogenesis and angiogenesis in a porcine heart model of myocardial infarction [332].

ANGIOMYOGENESIS

In the angiomyogenesis study, the human myoblasts were transduced with retroviral and adenoviral vectors carrying Lac-Z and human VEGF$_{165}$ genes, respectively. The cells were characterized for VEGF$_{165}$ transduction and expression efficiency by immunostaining, ELISA, immunoblotting and RT-PCR.

A porcine heart model of infarction was created in eight female swines by left circumflex artery ligation. The animals were grouped as control and myoblast-implanted. Angiography was performed to ensure complete occlusion of the blood vessel. Infarction was confirmed with MIBI-Tc^{99}m SPECT scanning. Four weeks later, 5ml basal DMEM without or with 3×10^8 human myoblasts carrying VEGF$_{165}$ and Lac-Z genes. The animals were maintained on cyclosporine (5 mg/kg body weight) for six weeks post-operatively. Hearts were then explanted and processed for immunocytochemical studies.

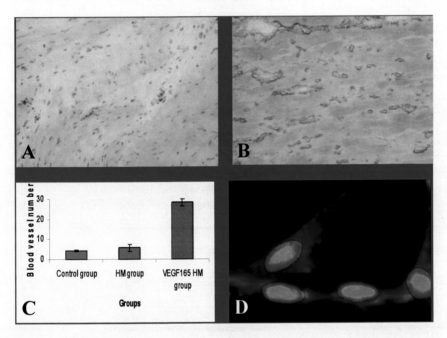

Figure 21. (a) Control infarcted myocardium immunostained for von Willebrand factor(vWF) VIII and counterstained with eosin to show capillaries and scar tissues. (b) VEGF $_{165}$transduced myoblasts produced increased vascular density, (c) seven times that of the control in the number of capillaries. (d) Immunofluorecent VEGF$_{165}$ myoblasts.

The transduction efficiency for Lac-Z and VEGF$_{165}$ was 75-80% and >95% respectively. The transduced myoblasts continued to secrete VEGF165 for longer than 18 days, at significantly higher level (37 ± 3ng/ml) than non-transduced ones (200 ± 30pg/ml). Dye exclusion test revealed >95% cell viability at the time of injection. Histological examination showed extensive survival of the grafted myoblasts expressing Lac-Z gene in and around the infarct. The SPECT scans showed improved perfusion in the infarcted region. Immunostaining for vWF-VIII expression showed significantly higher number (28.3 ± 1.8) of microvessels in the infarction region after transplantation of hVEGF$_{165}$ transduced myoblasts as compared to the DMEM injected (4.2 ± 0.4) pig hearts at low power (200x/field) (Figure 21C).

Most previous studies to achieve therapeutic angiogenesis have relied on a single growth factor protein or its gene administration. Angiogenesis involves interplay between numerous growth factors, their receptors, and intracellular signals. Recent studies have focused on the use of a combination of factors or their genes. The synergistic interaction in vivo between VEGF$_{165}$ and Ang-1 to produce functional and leak-resistant neovascularization support the suitability of their combined administration. Combining the synergistic effect between VEGF$_{165}$ and Ang-1, together with myoblast therapy, has the additional advantage of inducing myogenesis together with angiogenesis for treatment of ischemic limbs [355]. The present study involved transduction of VEGF$_{165}$ and Ang-1 genes into autologous skeletal myoblasts using a new bicistronic adenoviral vector for the treatment of hind limb ischemia in a rabbit model.

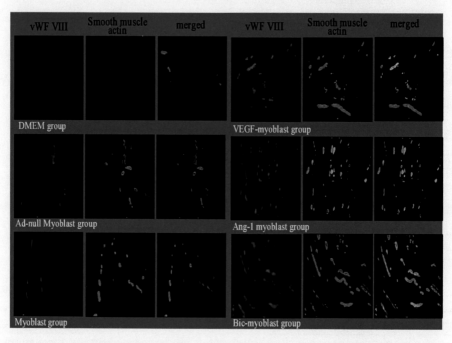

Figure 22. Neovascularization of infracted myocardia at 12 weeks after treatment. When compared to the DMEM group, both the ad-null myoblast group and the non-transduced myoblast group showed formation of new capillaries. These latters are less numerous and less mature than the transduced myoblast groups.

Unlike the use of monocistronic vectors, bicistronic vector provides a less cumbersome delivery option by simplifying the construct design and enabling delivery of the two transgenes in a single administration [356]. Although the donor myoblasts survived adequately in vivo for 6 weeks or longer, as assessed with X-gal staining, mortality was still inadvertent, despite use of autologous cells. Similar to previous findings, the fate of our implanted myoblasts was either that they fused to mature fibers of the host, to regenerating muscle cells of the host, or to other implanted myoblasts, they remained quiescent as mononucleated cells, or they died [357,358].

The donor myoblasts transduced with Ad-Bic is simultaneously expressed both VEGF and Ang-1, and significantly increased neovascularization in the ischemic porcine myocardium (Figure 22). Double fluorescent immunostaining of tissue sections for vWF and SMA revealed that a large proportion of the vessels observed were coated with smooth muscle layer. This observation is in agreement with previous studies that show the role of Ang-1 in development of mature, stable, non-leaky vessels [359]. This suggests that increased blood vessel density was genuinely the result of Ad-Bicis transduced myoblasts treatment.

FIRST IN MAN (FIM) STUDIES

Myoblast Autograft

On May 14, 2002, a 55-year-old man suffering acute ischemic myocardial infarction received cGMP-produced pure myoblasts into his beating myocardium as an adjunct to off-pump coronary artery bypass grafting (CABG). Professor Eugene Sim of the National University Hospital of Singapore led his team in the operation.

Coronary angiography previously demonstrated a right dominant system, 80% occlusion of the mid-left anterior descending artery, 70% occlusion of the proximal first diagonal branch and 50% stenosis of the circumflex artery. The mid-right coronary artery was occluded with good collateral supply from the left coronary artery. Echocardiography 5 days later revealed akinetic apex, anterior wall and septum of the left ventricle, with a left ventricular ejection fraction of 31%.

Tomographic Tc99m tetrofosmin scan 25 days after the acute myocardial infarction revealed a large partially reversible defect on the anterior wall and a moderate-sized reversible defect on the inferior wall. After qualifying for the inclusion/exclusion criteria, signing patients' informed consent, and obtaining approval from the hospital ethics committee, the patient was included as a volunteer for myocardial cell transplantation adjunct to CABG at 2 months after the initial presentation.

Approximately 2.5g of rectus femoris muscle biopsy was taken under local anesthesia from the patient and cultured under cGMP for 32 days to produce one billion cells. Myoblast purity of >99% was ascertained by positive immunostain for human desmin.

Under direct vision and stabilization with the Octopus III tissue stabiliser, 4.65×10^8 autologous myoblasts in 3 mL serum were injected into the myocardium within 15 minutes using a 27-gauge needle. Twenty-five injections were made on the anterior wall, near the apex, on the posterior wall, in and around the infarcted areas. These injections of 0.1 mL to 0.2 mL each were performed at half- to one-minute intervals to observe for dysrhythmias.

The patient recovered well from the operation. Serum creatine kinase was 222 µg/L and the MB fraction was 6 µg/L at 3 hours post-operatively, and 385 µg/L and 6 µg/L respectively at 12 hours. Postoperative 24-hour Holter monitoring revealed no arrhythmia. The patient was discharged on the eighth post-operative day.

His EKG has shown no arrhythmia. He has shown good effort tolerance, no dyspnea or angina, and a significant increase in ejection fraction since three weeks post-operatively. This case study suggests that beating-heart cellular cardiomyoplasty can be a safe and viable option.

Myoblast Allograft

Myoblast allograft is being developed to prevent and to alleviate heart muscle degeneration [348]. We report its *first application in man.*

The feasibility and safety of myoblast allograft was assessed by injecting the infarcted myocardia of two men, aged 63 and 49, with 1.1 and 1.2 billion myoblasts respectively, using 2-month cyclosporine immunosuppression.

Donor myoblasts were manufactured in compliance with current Good Manufacture Practice (cGMP) and ISO 9001 conditions. About 2.18g of muscle biopsy was taken under local anesthesia from the rectus femoris of a 20 year-old pathogen-free male volunteer, after he had met muscle donor criteria and had signed informed consent. At harvest, the culture yielded 3.64×10^9 myoblasts that were 98.3% pure by positive desmin immunostain. It was 91.5% viable according to vital dye exclusion tests. The cells were potent in myogenecity in that myotubes comprised more than 99% of the culture in fusion medium. Throughout the culture and for the final injectates, the myoblasts were free of endotoxin, mycoplasma, and negative for sterility (14 day test) and gram stain (absence of gram positive or negative bacteria) according to certified laboratory analyses.

Both patients enrolled as clinical trial subjects after qualifying for inclusion/exclusion criteria, signing patients' informed consents, and obtaining institutional and academy approval. They had atherosclerosis, coronary artery disease, history of acute myocardial infarction, stable angina Functional Class IV (CCS), and arterial hypertension II (risk 4). Positron emission tomography (PET) with 18FDG revealed scarred myocardium in LV septal, apical, and anterior/posterior wall regions. Echocardiography showed regional akinesis/hypokinesis, LVEF being 41% and 38% for the subjects respectively. Single-photon emission computed tomography (SPECT) with 30 mCi ^{99}mTc-tetrofosmin was performed during exercise with bicycle and during rest. Ischaemic changes and scars were confirmed, with significant perfusion defective areas (Figures 23, 24). Total LVEF were 39% and 38% for the two subjects respectively. Coronarography revealed calcination, stenosis, and occlusion of the left and right coronary arteries. Left ventriculography demonstrated hypokinesis in segments II, III, IV, and V in the older subject.

Our 15 years of experience of injecting allogenic myoblasts into 280 muscular dystrophy patients and 31 years of animal allograft/xenograft studies suggested that eight weeks of cyclosporine immunosuppression are sufficient to allow foreign myoblast engraftment in heart patients. The subjects took two oral doses of cyclosporine totaling 5 to 7 mg/kg body weight per day, beginning at five days before grafting, weaning at half-doses in the last two weeks, and off cyclosporine at eight weeks after grafting. Whole blood trough level of cyclosporine was monitored every three days at 23 hours after the morning dose. Doses were adjusted to maintain the level at about 250 ng/mL.

Academician Leo A. Bockeria of the Russian Academy of Medical Sciences is the world's first to have injected the hearts of the patients with allogenic myoblasts. On January 17, 2003, the subjects underwent bypass grafting immediately prior to myoblast implantation. They received 18/19 injections totaling 1.1/1.2 billion myoblasts respectively. The 10-min procedure was performed open-chest on an ice-chilled, non-beating heart with the subject under general anesthesia and on respirator. Cells were injected at 100×10^6 /mL. The 0.5 mL injections were made under direct vision between the infarcted and viable myocardium, and into scarred tissue.

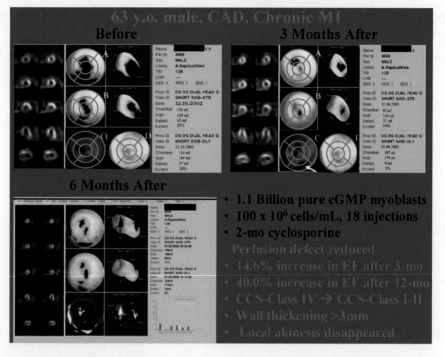

Figure 23. Polar views on PET and SPECT tomograms of the left ventricular myocardium before and at 3 and 6 months after myoblast allograft for the 63 y.o. patient. Before surgery (a) 35% perfusion defect during exercise and (b) 20% at rest, (c) significant decrease of systolic thickening and (d) preserved metabolism are indicative of scarred and hibernated myocardium. After surgery (a) 14% perfusion defect during exercise and (b) 5% at rest, (c) decrease in systolic thickening is less, and perfusion in the posterior wall (arrow) has been retrieved. (d) Metabolism is preserved and shows no change.

The subjects recovered from the general anesthesia with no rash or fever. Holter EKG monitor registered sporadic ventricular arrhythmias and ventricular extrasystoles that were eventually eliminated with Amiodarone treatment. Both patients were discharged after careful observation for 3 weeks. There was no evidence of overt blood pressure changes or renal failure.

Despite cyclosporine discontinuation at 2 months postoperatively, no sign of rejection was observed. At 3, 6 and 9-month follow-ups, both subjects were in stable condition at Class I-II (CCS). They no longer suffered angina or shortness of breath. Echocardiography showed significant increases in LVEF respectively with no local akinetic/hypokinetic regions. SPECT with [30] mCi 99mTc-tetrofosmin confirmed similar LVEF increases and demonstrated reduction on perfusion defective areas during exercise and rest (Figures 23, 24). [18]FDG accumulation was equable throughout LV myocardium, and glucose metabolism changes were not revealed.

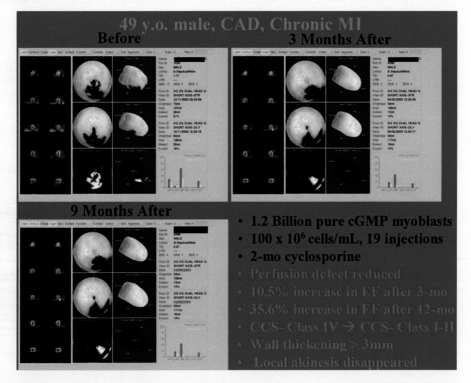

Figure 24. Polar views on PET and SPECT tomograms of the left ventricular myocardium before and at 3 and 9 months after myoblast allograft for the 49 y.o. patient showing similar improvement with time.

Human myoblast allografts may provide an alternative therapy for heart muscle degeneration and prevention of heart attack, with virtually unlimited cell availability and only 2-month immunosuppression. Cell potency from young donors is much higher than that of autografts from older heart patients. The regenerative heart is also a rejuvenated heart. Whereas good cells are readily available from cell banks in allografts, autograft patients have to be biopsied and wait about one month for their own myoblasts to grow to reach one billion in number. In acute myocardial infarction, the immediate allografts may prevent fibroblast infiltration and eventual scar formation.

Patients with infectious diseases such as AIDS can be treated with allografts without fear of contamination of the cell culture system [348,351,352].

Furthermore, heart patients with genetic diseases such as the muscular dystrophies can be treated with genetically normal allografts.

The survival of the two subjects without any sign of rejection after cyclosporine withdrawal confirmed our report on safety in the human/porcine cardiac xenografts [348,351,352]. Cyclosporine immunosuppression for 3 months allowed allogeneic myoblasts to survive, develop, and function in a muscle of a Duchenne muscular dystrophy patient, expressing the therapeutic protein dystrophin at 3 months [256] unto 6 years [262] after myoblast transfer. Myoblast autograft has been demonstrated to have survived and developed up to 17.5 months after implantation [319,369] in an ischaemic heart patient. The myoblast purity of this study was determined using CD56+, an antibody which reacts with stem cells, neurons, and fibroblasts rather than with myoblasts. CD56+ antibody yields false data on myoblast purity.

Clinical Trials to Date (Nov. 2003)   NTR = no test report on cGMP

START DATE	TEAM	TYPE of TRIAL	TOTAL NO. OF SUBJECTS	TOTAL NO. OF SURVIVALS	CELLS / TESTS	RESULTS	REFERENCE
6/15/00	Menasche / Paris	Open heart with bypass, autograft	11 patients	10	$(0.5-1.2B) \times 10^9$, 65% pure, 95% viable, NTR	EF from 25% to 35%, donor cells survived, function improved	Lancet, 2001 Lancet, 2002
5/23/01	Smits/Bioheart (Rotterdam, Milan, Mt. Sinai)	Endovascular, autograft	24 patients	20	$25\text{-}300 \times 10^6$, 35% - 90% pure, NTR	4 died; >50% patients developed arrhythmis	Am J Cardiol 92 supp (6), 2003
5/30/01	Dib / Diacrin, (Ariz HI/ Ohio State U., Cleveland Clinic UCLA)	Open heart with bypass, autograft	12 patients	12	10, 30, 100, 300 millions, 35-95% pure, NTR	EF from 22% to 34%, wall thickening, gap junction , no connexin 34, 4 Patients had arrhythmia before & after procedure	Am J Cardiol 92 supp (6), 2003
5/14/02	Law/Sim/NUH, Singapore	Open heart with bypass, autograft	1 patient	1	0.46×10^9, 98% pure, 95% potent, all cGMP tests completed	EF 31% to 34%; NYHA Level III to II	Handbook of Cardiovascular Cell Transplantation, Ch 17, 2003 Am J Cardiol 92 supp (6), 2003 J Mol Med, 2003
1/17/03	Law/ Bockeria/ Russian Academy of Medical Sciences	Open heart with bypass, allograft	2 patients	2	1×10^9, 98% pure, 80% viable, 95% potent, all cGMP tests completed	EF 39% to 47%; CCS III/IV to CS I; LV Defective area reduced, wall thickening.	Handbook of Cardiovascular Cell Transplantation, Ch 17, 2003 Am J Cardiol 92 supp (6), 2003 J Mol Med, 2003
2001	Hosp. Avellaneda	Surgery, autograft	1 patient	1	NTR	Unknown	BAM 13:17, 2003
2002	Siminiak / Poland	Open heart with bypass, autograft	10 patients	9	20 millions; NTR	EF 28% to 35%, wall thickening	Am J Cardiol 92 supp (6), 2003
2002	Canalejo/Univ. Navarra	Surgery, autograft	10 patients	Unknown	NTR	No adverse reaction	BAM 13:17, 2003
2003	Kao/ Nanjing U.	Surgery, autograft	3 patients	Unknown	NTR	Unknown	BAM 13:17, 2003

Figure 25. Phase I clinical trials of myoblasts for heart muscle degeneration.

Including those studied recently in the Magic trial, more than 150 patients have received myoblasts worldwide since the initial procedure in June 2000

(Figure 24). Mortality has been less than 10%. If future myoblast allografts prove to be safe and efficacious in treating heart dysfunction, the 2-month immunosuppression, when compared to life-long immunosuppression in heart transplant patients, will greatly improve life expectancy and quality of life of heart patients. Moreover, myoblast allografts can significantly reduce medical cost considering quality control and analysis tests on one lot of 50 billion myoblasts are much less costly than the same tests on 50 lots of one billion myoblasts. Future allograft studies are warranted. The cessation of akinesis/hypokinesis, reduction in perfusion defects, and increase in LVEF suggest that future myoblast allograft studies are warranted.

The future of HCT lies with myoblast allograft, 90% delivered endovascularly and 10% epicardially in adjunct to CABG. Myoblasts will likely be transduced with $VEGF_{165}$, Ang-1,TGF-β, or similar factors to allow concomitant angiomyogenesis.

Our ongoing clinical trial is based on unequivocal evidence of cGMP-produced pure human myoblasts and proof of concept for Heart Cell Therapy. Human myoblasts survived and integrated into porcine ischemic myocardium, allowing concomitant cell therapy and gene therapy to produce angiomyogenesis. Whereas the newly formed myofibers harbor satellite cells and impart regenerative capacity to the heart muscle, the genetic transformation of cardiomyocytes in vivo to become regenerative heterokaryons through myoblast genome transfer [328] constitutes the ultimate heart repair. The regenerative heart [349] also contains trans-differentiated cardiomyocytes of myoblastic origin. In all three scenarios, new contractile filaments are deposited to improve heart contractility. This latter can be translated into the improvement in the quality of life of heart patients and in the prevention of heart attacks.

It can be concluded that pure myoblasts transduced with Ang-1 and $VEGF_{165}$, when injected intramyocardially, are potential therapeutic transgene vehicles for concurrent angiogenesis and myogenesis to treat heart failure [348,350]. Immunosuppression using cyclosporine for six weeks is effective for long-term survival of xenografts or allografts. The feasibility and preliminary safety/efficacy observed in the world's first human myoblast allografts lead the way in developing a low-cost, easy-to-use treatment for heart failure and prevention of heart attacks, with virtually unlimited cell availability and short-term immunosuppression.

Chapter IV

THE WORLD'S FIRST MYOBLAST STUDY OF TYPE II DIABETIC PATIENTS

Type II diabetes, also called non-insulin-dependent diabetes mellitus (NIDDM), is characterized by high blood glucose resulting from the genetic defect of the GLUT4 genome. The latter is manifested in the diminished glucose uptake into skeletal muscles. In normal human beings, insulin combines with insulin receptors to change the membrane conformation of skeletal muscle fibers, allowing blood glucose to move down its concentration gradient into the fibers for metabolism.

A disorder called 'insulin resistance' exists in Type II diabetic patients in which normal or even elevated levels of plasma insulin would not elicit normal glucose uptake into the muscle fibers. This study hypothesizes that these diabetic fibers exhibit less insulin receptors, or that these receptors exhibit abnormal molecular conformation, or both. Considering that highly metabolic muscle fibers constitute more than 50% of the human body by volume and weight, failure of blood glucose to gain entry would undoubtedly lead to high blood glucose and result in various organ failures sequentially.This is not the only defect, but it is likely the primary and significant one.

A potential genetic treatment of the disease involves myoblast transfer therapy (MTT) which is a platform technology of cell transplantation, genome therapy and tissue engineering [326,328]. It consists of culturing immature muscle cells called myoblasts, derived originally from a 2g skeletal muscle biopsy from a healthy, young, male donor, and implanting them into the major muscle groups of the upper and lower extremities of the diabetic patients.

The myoblasts exhibit natural cell fusion, and transfer their nuclei carrying the normal human genome into the host skeletal muscle fibers to achieve genetic repair. Others fuse among themselves to form new myofibers that exhibit normal insulin receptors of donor origin. Through both mechanisms, new insulin receptors of donor origin that are genetically normal, will be produced in the skeletal myofibers of the host.

The survival, development, and functioning of the implanted allogeneic myoblasts have previously been demonstrated in studies involving about 260 muscular dystrophy subjects and two chronically myocardial infracted heart subjects with 100% safety and substantial efficacy results [349,351]. Immunorejection was minimized using two months of cyclosporine following MTT. In addition, over 120 ischemic heart patients have received autologous myoblasts in their hearts in 10 countries. Mortality rate has been less than 10% traversing the last four years, with efficacy data being collected in Phase II clinical trials in Europe. Reported here are the world's first genetic transplants of two Type II diabetic patients using allogeneic myoblasts.

Human myoblasts were manufactured according to the standard operating procedures (SOPs) of Cell Transplants Singapore Pte Ltd (CTS) with US patent no. 5,130,141 and Singapore patent no. 34490 (WO 96/18303) licenses. Cell production was in compliance with current good manufacturing practice (cGMP) and international organization for standardization (ISO) standard 9001 conditions. Around 2g of muscle biopsy was taken under local anesthesia from a 20-year-old, pathogen-free, male volunteer after he had met muscle donor criteria. Initial dissociation isolated approximately 10,000 satellite cells, which were then cultured accordingly to CTS's SOPs.

The culture yielded 47.4×10^9 myoblasts that were 100% pure by positive desmin immunostain, and 92.8% viable according to vital dye exclusion tests. The cells were potent in myogenecity in that numerous myotubes were observed within four days in a fusion medium. Throughout the culture and for the final injectates, the myoblasts were free of endotoxin (<1.0EU/ml) and mycoplasma, and negative for sterility (14-day test) and gram stain (absence of gram positive or negative bacteria) according to certified laboratory analyses outside CTS.

Patient 1 is 42 years old, 157cm tall, and weighs 68kg. Patient 2 is 36 years old, 158cm tall, and also weighs 68kg. Diagnosis showed about two years history of Type II diabetes and hypertension but otherwise normal in heart, lung, kidney, and liver function without obesity. The laboratory report revealed tests results for syphilis, hepatitis B surface antigens, antibodies to HIV and hepatitis C virus to be negative.

Both patients had previously been enrolled as clinical trial subjects after qualifying for inclusion/exclusion criteria, and signing patients' informed consents with institutional approval. The subjects took two oral doses of cyclosporine totalling 5–7mg/kg body weight per day, beginning two days before grafting, weaning at half-dosage in the last two weeks, and off cyclosporine at eight weeks after grafting. The whole blood trough level of cyclosporine was monitored every two weeks. Doses were adjusted in an attempt to maintain the level at about 250ng/ml.

Myoblasts were harvested and processed under biological safety cabinets (Class 100) inside a cleanroom. Having been washed thoroughly, they were suspended in the injection medium. Quality assurance/quality control processes ensued, and the final quality control release testforms were issued for each of the two subjects. The myoblasts were then carried in syringes within sterile enclosures into two surgical suites for simultaneous implantation into both subjects. These were the world's first cases of allogeneic myoblasts being injected into Type II diabetic patients.

The patients received 132 injections each and 24/23.4 billion myoblasts, respectively.The two hour procedure was performed with the patients under general anesthesia. Cells were injected at 50×10^6/ml and the injections were made under direct vision into 54 major muscle groups of each subject. The patients were transferred to the intensive care unit, where they recovered from the anesthesia and routine monitors were administered.

The subjects recovered from the general anesthesia without rash or fever, and both patients were discharged at 48 hours post-operatively.

Most pertinent to the specific goal of this study was that, despite cyclosporine discontinuation at two months postoperatively, no sign of rejection was observed. The patients appear to have good general health before and after MTT. Plasma glucose and insulin levels data were collected.

This pioneering feasibility/safety study of myoblast allografts into the skeletal muscles of Type II diabetic patients leads the way in developing a genetic treatment for the disease [360]. The immunosuppressant cyclosporine used in this study is known to increase plasma glucose. The subjects were weaned off cyclosporine. They will be further monitored to determine the preliminary efficacy, if any, of the 24-billion PMGT. Meanwhile, the procedure appears to be safe for both subjects.

Chapter V

FUTURE PERSPECTIVES

ESSENCE OF CELL THERAPY

The cell is the basic unit of all lives. It is that infinitely small entity which life is made of. With the immense wisdom and knowledge of the human race, we have not been able to produce a living cell from nonliving ingredients such as DNA, ions, and biochemicals.

Cell Culture is the only method known to man for the replication of cells in vitro. With proper techniques and precautions, normal cells can be cultured in sufficient quantity to repair, and to replenish degenerates and wounds [361].

Cell transplantation bridges the gap between in vitro and in vivo systems, and allows propagation of "new life" in degenerative tissues or organs of the living yet genetically defective or injured body.

Cell fusion transfers all the normal genes within the nucleus like delivering a repair kit to the abnormal cell. It is important to recognize that, for proper installation and future operation, the software packaged in the chromosomes needs other cell organelles as hardware to operate.

Correction of a gene defect occurs spontaneously at the cellular level after cell fusion. The natural integration, regulation and expression of the full complement of over 30,000 normal genes impart the normal phenotypes onto the heterokaryon. Protein(s) or factor(s) that were not produced by the host genome because of the genetic defect are now produced by the donor genome that is normal. Various cofactors derived from expression of the other genes corroborate to restore the normal phenotype.

HEART MUSCLE GENES

The development of CardioChip [347] allows early diagnosis of cardiovascular diseases using 10,368 expressed sequence tags (ESTs). In collaboration with Prof. C C Liew of Harvard University, heart muscle genes can be identified to provide the template for early diagnosis (Figures 26, 27). Subjects so identified can have muscle biopsy taken before any symptom occurs. Myoblasts can be processed and deposited in a cell bank for future transduced HMGT to prevent sudden heart attack.

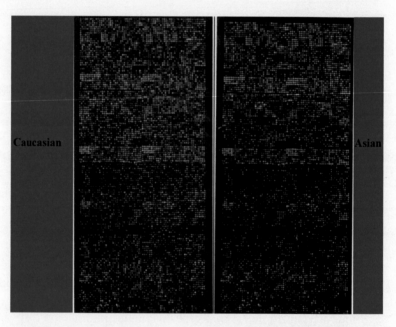

Figure 26. CardioChip analyses of Caucacian and Asian myoblast ESTs to determine 1) if there are any contaminants, 2) the consistency of myoblast production by the American team vs the Singapore team, 3) the myogenic genome for the heart.

THE ULTIMATE GENE TRANSFER

The use of myoblasts as gene transfer vehicles dates as early as 1978.1 In mammals, myoblasts is the only cell type which divides extensively, migrates, fuses naturally to form syncytia, loses MHC-1 antigens soon after fusion, and develops to occupy 50% of the body weight in humans. These combined properties render myoblasts ideal for gene transfer.

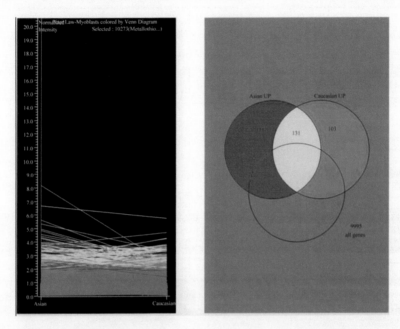

Figure 27. CardioChip analyses of Caucacian and Asian myoblasts identified 78 ESTs related to heart muscle in its early development. These ESTs can be used as a template for early diagnosis of heart muscle diseases.

Natural transduction of normal nuclei ensures orderly replacement of dystrophin and related proteins at the cellular level in DMD. This ideal gene transfer procedure is unique to muscle. After all, only myoblasts can fuse and only muscle fibers are multinucleated in the human body. By harnessing these intrinsic properties, MTT transfers all normal genes to achieve genetic repair. Since donor myoblasts also fuse among themselves to form normal fibers in MTT, the muscles benefit from the addition of genetically normal cells as well.

This differs significantly from the gene therapy format in which single copies of the down-sized dystrophin gene are transduced as viral conjugates into the mature dystrophic myofibers in which many proteins, both structural and regulatory, are lost. Multiple gene insertion is necessary to produce the lost proteins for the development of a cure or a treatment. More gene insertion is needed to produce the cofactors to regulate and to express these lost proteins in order to repair the degenerating cell.

CONTROLLED CELL FUSION

It will be useful to be able to control, initiate or facilitate cell fusion once myoblasts are injected. Myoblasts fuse readily at low serum concentration in culture [362]. The process is more complex in the in vivo situation.

As the myoblasts are injected intramuscularly into the extracellular matrix (ECM), injection trauma causes the release of basic fibroblast growth factor (bFGF) and large chondroitin-6-sulfate proteoglycan (LC6SP) [363]. These latter growth factors stimulate myoblast proliferation. Unfortunately, they also stimulate the proliferation of fibroblasts that are already present in increased amount in the dystrophic or the infarcted muscles. That is why it is necessary to inject as pure as possible fractions of myoblasts in MTT without contaminating fibroblasts.

Controlled cell fusion can be achieved by artificially increasing the concentration of LC6SP over the endogenous level. In addition, insulin or insulin-like growth factor I (IGF-1) [364] may facilitate the developmental process, resulting in the formation of myotubes soon after myoblast injection. The use of bFGF, LC6SP and IGF-1 at optimal concentrations in the cell culture medium and in the injection medium will be examined.

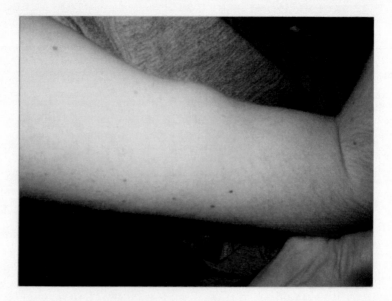

Figure 28. HMGT enhances the size, shape, consistency and strength of a biceps brachii muscle in the upper arm of a patient suffering Infantile Facioscapulohumeral Dystrophy.

ANTI-AGING COSMETIC ENHANCEMENT

HMGT can significantly contribute to the field of gerontology and plastic surgery. With cell therapy, implantation of silicone could be avoided. The use of fat cells could be used in a much more natural way to replace silicone injections for facial, breast and hip augmentation. Myotubes are known to survive in adipose tissues [365]. Modified adipose tissue involving mixing and/or hybridization of myoblasts and fat cells can be used to control size, shape and consistency of body parts. Since muscle cells do not break down as easily as fat cells, good results may be long-lasting. Today, body builders are in search of increasing muscle mass at the right places. The use of myoblast transfer to boost muscle mass is a natural solution.

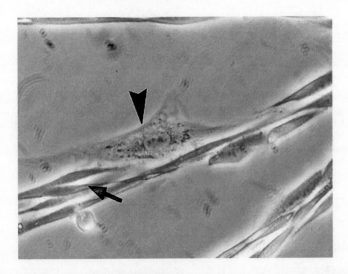

Figure 29. Myoblasts are small, spindle-shaped cells that can survive and develop in intercellular fluid without blood supply. Fibroblasts are coarse, polygonal cells that have shorter life.

By now, the survival, development and functioning of donor myoblasts in host muscles, either normal or scarred, have been repeatedly demonstrated by numerous laboratories. HMGT can thus modulate the size, shape, consistency and strength of all external body parts (Figure 28). Since myoblasts are small (8 to 15 µm)/ spindle-shaped / durable cells when compared to the relatively large/ polygonal/ rough skin fibroblasts (Figure 29), myoblasts can be "plated" over diseased /degenerative/old skins to cover wrinkles/blemishes/spot (Figure 30). The angiomyogenic HMGT will not only treat heart infarcts, but should also have application to sexual impotency, baldness, red lips and pink faces by providing more muscles, blood supplies and nutrients. This on-going development promises anti-aging aesthetica for health and beauty, and shall highly increase the quality of life of mankind.

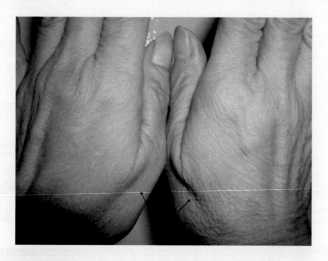

Figure 30. The left hand of a 60-yr-old female worker appeared "younger" with lighter tone and less wrinkles 2 weeks after external application of one billion allogeneic myoblasts without immunosuppression. The right hand received equal volume and number of application of the carrier solution.

BONE DEGENERATION

During embryonic development, mesenchymal progenitor cells differentiate into myoblasts, osteoblasts, chondrocytes, adipocytes, fibroblasts and cardiomyocytes under controls of various regulatory factors. Ectopic bone formation in muscle has been achieved through implantation of bone morphogenetic protein (BMP). BMP-2 was shown to convert the differentiation pathway of clonal myoblasts into the osteoblast lineage [245]. Our combined use of BMP-2, myoblasts and hydroxyapetite produced bone formation to fill a small hole drilled on a rabbit skull (Figure 31). This opens new ways to treat conditions of bone degeneration such as the degeneration of tooth pulp, hip, bone/joint, and long bone fractures. Given the ability to mass-produce myoblasts that can be transformed into osteoblasts, and potentially chondrocytes, the difficulty of proliferating osteoblasts and chondrocytes can be overcome. Cultured autologous chondrocytes can be used to repair deep cartilage defects in the femorotibial articular surface of the human knee joint [218].

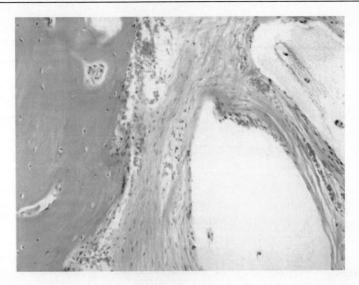

Figure 31. A combination of human myoblasts, BMP-2 and hydoxyappetite produced bone-like filling for a minute hole drilled on the skull of a rabbit (left). Without myoblasts, only fibroblasts infiltrated a control hole filled with BMP-2 and hydoxyappetite.

MYOBLAST: THE UNIVERSAL GENE TRANSFER VEHICLES

Whereas MTT results in the formation of genetic mosaicism with gene transfer occurring in vivo, the production of heterokaryons in vitro has immense medical application. This can be achieved by controlled cell fusion with myoblasts.

This original program of research relates to the in culturo transfer of the normal nuclei with all of their normal genes from donor myoblasts into the genetically normal and/or abnormal cells, e.g. the cardiomyocytes. This development is especially important considering that cardiomyopathic symptoms develop in mid adolescence in about 10% of the DMD population [20]. By age 18, all DMD individuals develop caridomyopathy [21]. Undoubtedly, the ability to replenish degenerated and degenerating cardiomyocytes will have immense impact on heart diseases even in the normal population [366] where there is a great shortage of hearts for transplantation.

Normal cardiomyocytes exhibit very limited ability to proliferate in vivo or in vitro. The heart muscles damaged in heart attacks or in hereditary cardiomyopathy cannot repair themselves through regeneration. The integration of the skeletal muscle cell characteristic, mitosis, will enable the heterkaryotic cardiomyocytes to proliferate in vitro.

Controlled cell fusion between normal myoblasts and normal cardiomyocytes may result in heterokaryons exhibiting the characteristics of both parental myogenic cell types. Clones can be selected based on their abilities to undergo mitosis in vitro, to develop desmosomes, gap junctions, and to contract strongly in synchrony after cell transplantation.

These genetically superior cells can then be delivered through catheter pathways after mapping of the injured sites. With the ability to grow large quantity of these cardiomyocytes, the correction of structural, electrical and contractile abnormalities in cardiomyopathy can be tested first in dystrophic, cardiomyopathic hamsters [367,368] and, if safe and effective, in humans.

The genetic transfer of the mitotic property of myoblasts onto cardiomyocytes with in vitro controlled cell fusion enables the resulting heterokaryotic cardiomyocytes to multiply, yielding enough number of cells for the cell transplant to be effective.

The use of myoblasts as gene transfer vehicles does not stop with myogenic cells. Myoblasts have been genetically modified to provide systemic delivery of human growth hormone [120,121] and may in time provide long-term secretion of insulin for diabetes and various hormones and/or factors. Myoblasts tranduced to secrete opiode derivatives may be used to treat pain, depression and addictions.

AUTOMATED CELL PROCESSORS

The great demand for normal myoblasts, myotubes and young muscles, the labor intensiveness and high cost of cell culturing, harvesting and packaging, and the fallibility of human imprecision will soon necessitate the invention and development of automated cell processors capable of producing huge quantities of viable, sterile, genetically well-defined and functionally demonstrated biologics, an example of which are the myogenic cells.

This invention will be one of the most important offspring of modern day computer science, mechanical engineering and cytogenetics (Figure 32). The intakes will be for biopsies of various human tissues. The computer will be programmed to process tissue(s), with precision controls in time, space, proportions of culture ingredients and apparatus maneuvers. Cell conditions can be monitored at any time during the process and flexibility is built-in to allow changes. Different protocols can be programmed into the software for culture, controlled cell fusion, harvest and package. The outputs supply injectable cells ready for cell therapy or shipment. The cell processor will be self-contained in a sterile enclosure large enough to house the hardware in which cells are cultured and manipulated. Various cell types can be manufactured depending on the software used.

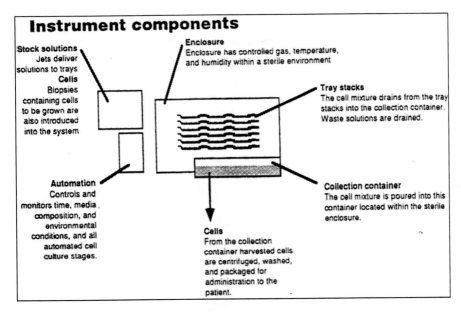

Figure 32. A basic design for the automated cell processor.

The automated cell processor will replace the current bulky inefficient culture equipment, elaborate manpower, and their mistakes. Its installation into clinics, hospitals and medical centers will allow customized medicine for individual patients by providing autologous HMGT. Fresh cells will be nearby. Cell costs will be reduced. Its contribution to human health is highly significant.

CELL THERAPY IS NOW

Health is the well-being of all body cells. In hereditary degenerative diseases, sick cells need repairing and dead cells need replacing for health maintenance.

Cell culture is the way to generate new, live cells that are capable of surviving, developing and functioning in the body after transplantation, replacing degenerated cells that are lost.

Myoblasts are the only cells in the body capable of natural cell fusion. The latter allows the transfer of all of the normal genes into genetically defective cells to achieve phenotypic repair through complementation. HMGT/MTT on DMD is the first human gene therapy demonstrated to be safe and effective. The use of HMGT/MTT to transfer any other genes and their promoters/enhancers to treat other forms of diseases is underway. Endogenous to the human body, myoblasts will prove to be efficient, safe and universal gene transfer vehicles. Since a foreign gene always exerts its effect on a cell, cell therapy will always be the common pathway to health. After all, cells are what life is made of.

REFERENCES

[1]   O'Rahilly R, Muller F. *Developmental stages in human embryos*. Meriden: Meriden-Stinehour Press, 1987:1-306.

[2]   Jacobson M. *Developmental neurobiology*. New York: Holt, Rinehart & Winston Inc, 1970:1-465.

[3]   Banker BQ, Przybylski RJ, Van der Meulen JP, Victor M, eds. *Research in muscle development and the muscle spindle*. Princeton: Excerpta Medica, 1971:1-226.

[4]   Pearson ML, Epstein HF, eds. *Muscle development. Molecular and cellular control*. New York: Cold Spring Harbor Laboratory, 1982:339-96, 509-67.

[5]   Davidson EH. *Gene activity in early development*. 2nd ed. New York: Academic Press, 1976:175-9.

[6]   McComas AJ. Neuromuscular function and disorders. Boston: Butterworths, 1977:1-364.

[7]   Hoffman, EP, Brown RH, Kunkel LM. Dystrophin: the protein product of the Duchenne muscular dystrophy locus. *Cell* 1987; 51:919-28.

[8]   Monaco AP, Neve RL, Colletti-Feener C et al. Isolation of candidate cDNAs for portions of the Duchenne muscular dystrophy gene. *Nature* 1986; 323:646-50.

[9]   Koenig M. Hoffman EP, Bertelson CJ et al. Complete cloning of the Duchenne muscular dystrophy (DMD) cDNA and preliminary genomic organization of the DMD gene in normal and affected individuals. *Cell* 1987; 50:509-17.

[10]   Brooke MH, Fenichel GM, Griggs RC, et al. Clinical investigation of Duchenne muscular dystrophy: interesting results in a trial of prednisone. *Arch Neurol* 1987; 44:812-7.

[11] Brooke MH, Fenichel GM, Griggs RC, et al. Clinical investigation in Duchenne dystrophy: 2: Determination of the "power" of therapeutic trials based on the natural history. *Muscle Nerve* 1983; 6:91-103.

[12] Fenichel GM, Florence JM, Pestronk A, et al. Long-term benefit from prednisone therapy in Duchenne muscular dystrophy. *Neurology* 1991; 41:1874-7.

[13] Fenichel GM, Mendell JR, Moxley RT, et al. A comparison of daily and alternate-day prednisone therapy in the treatment of Duchenne muscular dystrophy. *Arch Neur* 1991; 48: 575-9.

[14] Mendell JR, Moxley RT, Griggs RC, et al. Randomized, double-blind six-month trial of prednisone in Duchenne's muscular dystrophy. *N Eng J Med* 1989; 320:1592-7.

[15] Stern LM, Fewings JD, Bretag AH, et al. The progression of Duchenne muscular dystrophy: clinical trial of allopurinol therapy. *Neurology* 1981; 31:422-6.

[16] Ziter FA, Allsop KG, Tyler FH. Assessment of muscle strength in Duchenne muscular dystrophy. *Neurology* 1977; 27:981-4.

[17] Walton JN, Gardner-Medwin D. Progressive muscular dystrophy and the myotonic disorders. In: Walton JN, Gardner-Medwin D, eds. *Disorders of voluntary muscle*. New York: Churchill Livingstone, 1981:487.

[18] Emery AE. Population frequencies of inherited neuromuscular diseases – a world survey. *Neuromuscular Disorders* 1991; 1:19.

[19] Iannaccone ST. Current status of Duchenne muscular dystrophy. *Ped Neurol* 1992; 39:879-94.

[20] Engel AG. Duchenne dystrophy. In: Banker BQ, Engel AG, eds. *Myology*. New York: McGraw Hill, 1986:1185.

[21] Nigro G, Comi LI, Politano L, et al. Treatment of cardiac involvement in late stage of Duchenne muscular dystrophy. *Acta Cardiomiologica* 1990; 2:13-24.

[22] Michelson AM, Russell ES, Harman PJ. Dystrophia muscularis: a hereditary primary myopathy in the house mouse. *Proc Nat Acad Sci* 1955; 41:1079-84.

[23] Meier H, West WT, Hoag WG. Preclinical histopathology of mouse muscular dystrophy. *Arch Path* 1965; 80:165-70.

[24] Law PK, Atwood HL. Nonequivalence of surgical and natural denervation in dystrophic mouse muscles. *Exp Neurol* 1972; 34:200-9.

[25] Law PK, Atwood HL, McComas AJ. Functional denervation in the soleus muscle of dystrophic mice. *Exp Neurol* 1976; 51:434-43.

[26] Mokri B, Engel AG. Duchenne dystrophy: electron microscopic findings pointing to a basic or early abnormality in the plasma membrane of the muscle fiber. *Neurology* 1975; 25:1111.

[27] Law PK, Saito A, Fleischer S. Ultrastructural changes in muscle and motor end-plate of the dystrophic mouse. *Exp Neurol* 1983; 80:361-82.

[28] Law PK, Cosmos E, Butler J, McComas AJ. The absence of dystrophic characteristics in normal muscles successfully cross-reinnervated by nerves of dystrophic genotype: physiological and cytochemical study of crosssed solei of normal and dystrophic parabiotic mice. *Exp Neurol* 1976; 51: 1-21.

[29] Law PK. "Myotrophic" influences on notoneurones of normal and dystrophic mice in parabiosis. *Exp Neurol* 1977; 54:444-52.

[30] Saito A, Law PK, Fleischer S. Study of neurotrophism with ultrastructure of normal/dystrophic parabiotic mice. *Muscle Nerve* 1983; 6:14-28.

[31] Carlson BM. A quantitative study of muscle fiber survival and regeneration in normal, predenervated, and Marcaine-treated free muscle grafts in the rat. *Exp Neurol* 1976; 52:421-32.

[32] Hakelius L, Nystrom B, Stalberg E. Histochemical and neurophysiological studies of autotransplanted cat muscle. *Scand J Plast Reconstr Surg* 1975;9:15- 24.

[33] Hall-Craggs ECB, Brand P. Effect of previous nerve injury on the regeneration of free autogenous muscle grafts. *Exp Neurol* 1977; 57:275-81.

[34] Mufti SA, Carlson BM, Maxwell LC, Faulkner JA. The free autografting of entire limb muscles in the cat: morphology. *Anat Rec* 1977; 188:417-30.

[35] Thompson N. A review of autogenous skeletal muscle grafts and their clinical applications. *Clin Plast Surg* 1974; 1:349-403.

[36] Studitsky AN. The restoration of muscle by means of transplantation of minced muscle tissue. *Dokl Akad Nauk SSSR* 1952; 84:389-92.

[37] Cosmos E. Muscle transplants: role in the etiology of herditary muscular dystrophy. In: Milhoart AP, ed. *Exploratory concepts in muscular dystrophy II*. Amsterdam: Excerpta Medica 1974:368-73.

[38] Carlson BM. The regeneration of skeletal muscle – a review. *Am J Anat* 1973; 137:119-50.

[39] Carlson BM. Regeneration of the completely excised gastrocnemius muscle in the frog and rat from minced muscle fragments. *J Morphol* 1968; 125:447-72.

[40] Allbrook D, Baker W de C, Kirkaldy-Willis WH. Muscle regeneration in experimental animals and in man. The cycle of tissue change that follows trauma in the injured limb syndrome. *J Bone Joint Surg* 1966; 48:153-69.

[41] Snow MH. Myogenic cell formation in regenerating rat skeletal muscle injured by mincing. I. A fine structural study. *Anat Rec* 1977; 188:181-200.

[42] Snow MH. Myogenic cell formation in regenerating rat skeletal muscle injured by mincing. II. An autoradiographic study. *Anat Rec* 1977; 188:201-18.

[43] Susheela AK, Hudgson P, Walton JN. Histological and histochemical studies of experimentally-induced degeneration and regeneration in normal and dystrophic mouse muscle. *J Neurol* 1969; 9:423-42.

[44] Mauro A. Satellite cells of skeletal muscle fibers. *J Biophys Biochem Cytol* 1961; 9:493-95.

[45] Carlson M, Hansen-Smith FM, Magon DK. The life history of a free muscle graft. In: Mauro A, ed. *Muscle Regeneration*. New York: Raven Press 1979:493-507.

[46] Cardasis CA, Cooper GW. A method for the chemical isolation of individual fibers and its application to a study of the effect of denervation on the number of nuclei per fiber. *J Exp Zool* 1975; 191:333-58.

[47] Burch T, Law PK. Normal development of muscle fibers and motor endplates in dystrophic mice. *Exp. Neurol. 58*:570–574, 1978

[48] Rowe RWD, Goldspink G. Muscle fiber growth in five different muscles in both sexes of mice. I. Normal mice. *J Anat* 1969; 104:519-30.

[49] Rowe RWD, Goldspink G. Muscle fiber growth in five different muscles in both sexes of mice. II. Dystrophic mice. *J Anat* 1969; 104:531-8.

[50] Law PK. Reduced regenerative capability of minced dystrophic mouse muscles. *Exp Neurol* 1978; 60:231-43.

[51] Mastaglia FL, Kakulas BA. Regeneration in Duchenne muscular dystrophy: a histological and histochemical study. *Brain* 1969; 92:809-18.

[52] Carlson BM, Gutmann E. Development of contractile properities of minced muscle regenerates in the rat. *Exp Neurol* 1972; 36:239-49.

[53] Church JCT. Cell populations in skeletal muscles after regeneration. *J Embryol Exp Morphol* 1970; 23:531-7.

[54] Vracko R, Benditt EP. Basal lamina: the scaffold for orderly cell replacement. *J Cell Biol* 1972; 55:406-19.

[55] Mufti SA. Regeneration following denervation of minced gastrocnemius muscle in mice. *J Neurol Sci* 1977; 33:251-66.

[56] Wakayama Y. Electron microscopic study on the satellite cells in the muscle of Duchenne muscular dystrophy. *J Neuropathol Exp Neurol* 1976; 35:532-40.

[57] Cosmos E. Muscle-nerve transplants. Experimental models to study influences on differentiation. *Physiologist* 1973; 16:167-77.

[58] Gallup B, Dubowitz V. Failure of "dystrophic" neurones to support functional regeneration of normal or dystrophic muscle in culture. *Nature* 1973; 243:287-9.

[59] Hironaka T, Miyata Y. Transplantation of skeletal muscle in normal and dystrophic mice. *Exp Neurol* 1975; 47:1-15.

[60] Laird JL, Timmer RF. Homotransplantation of dystrophic and normal muscle. *Arch Pathol* 1965; 80:442-6.

[61] Salafsky B. Functional studies of regenerated muscles from normal and dystrophic mice. *Nature* 1971; 229:270-2.

[62] Guth L, Yellin H. The dynamic nature of the so-called "fiber types" of mammalian skeletal muscle. *Exp Neurol* 1971; 31:277-300.

[63] Gutmann E, Schiaffino S, Hanzlikova V. Mechanism of compensatory hypertrophy in skeletal muscle of the rat. *Exp Neurol* 1971: 31:451-64.

[64] Ianuzzo CD, Gollnick PD, Armstrong RB. Compensatory adaptations of skeletal muscle fiber types to a long-term functional overload. *Life Sci* 1976; 19:1517-24.

[65] Vrbova G. The effect of motoneurone activity on the speed of contraction of striated muscle. *J Physiol (Lond)* 1963; 169:513-26.

[66] Bergel DH, Brown MC, Butler RG, Zacks RM. The effect of stretching a contracting muscle on its subsequent performance during shortening. *J Physiol (Lond)* 225:21-2P.

[67] Goldspink G, Tabary C, Tabary JC, et al. Effect of denervation on the adaptation of sarcomere number and muscle extensibility to the functional length of the muscle. *J Physiol (Lond)* 1974; 236:733-42.

[68] Tomanck RJ. A histochemical study of postnatal differentiation of skeletal muscle with reference to functional overload. *Dev Biol* 1974; 42:305-14.

[69] Yellin H. Changes in fiber types of the hypertrophying denervated hemidiaphragm. *Exp Neurol* 1974; 42:412-28.

[70] Eisen A, Karpati G, Carpenter S, Danon J. The motor unit profile of the rat soleus in experimental myopathy and reinnervation. *Neurology* 1974; 24:878-84.

[71] Liberman AR. The axon reaction: a review of the principal features of perikaryal responses to axon injury. *Int Rev Neurobiol* 1971; 14:49-124.

[72] Mark RF. Matching muscles and motoneurones. A review of some experiments on motor nerve regeneration. *Brain Res* 1969; 14:245-54.

[73] Law PK, Caccia MR. Physiological estimates of the sizes and numbers of motor units in soleus muscles of dystrophic mice. *J Neurol Sci* 1975; 24:251-6.

[74] Anderson, CW (ed). *Genetic Interaction and Gene Transfer*. New York: Brookhaven National Lab, 1978.

[75] Constantini F, Jacnisch R (eds). *Genetic Manipulation of the Early Mammalian Embryo Banbury Report 20*. New York: Cold Spring Harbor Lab, 1985.

[76] Friedmann T. *Gene Therapy – Fact and Fiction in Biology's New Approaches to Disease.* New York: Cold Spring Harbor Lab, 1983.

[77] Hogan, BLM, Constantini F, Lacy E (eds). *Manipulating the Mouse Embryo*. New York: Cold Spring Harbor Lab, 1986.

[78] Orkin SH. Reverse genetics and human diseases. *Cell* 1986; 47:845-50.

[79] Worton RG, Duff C, Sylvester TE, et al. Duchenne muscular dystrophy involving translocation of the DMD gene next to ribosomal RNA genes. *Science* 1984; 224:1447-1449.

[80] Kunkel LM, Hoffman EP. Duchenne/Becker muscular dystrophy: an overview of the gene, the protein and current diagnostics. *Med Bull* 1989; 45:630-43.

[81] Harley HG, Brook JD, Rundle SA, et al. Expansion of an unstable DNA region and phenotypic variation in myotonic dystrophy. *Nature* 1992; 355:545-7.

[82] Buxton J, Shelbourne P, Davies J, et al. Detection of an unstable fragment of DNA specific to individuals with myotonic dystrophy. *Nature* 1992; 355:547-8.

[83] Aslandis C, Jansen G, Amemiya C, et al. Cloning of the essential myotonic dystrophy region and mapping of the putative defect. *Nature* 1992; 355:548-51.

[84] Wijmenga C, Frantz R, Brouwer OF, et al. Location of facioscapulohumeral muscular dystrophy gene on chromosome 4. *Lancet* 1990; 336:651-3.

[85] Beckmann J, Richard I, Hillaire D, et al. *A gene for limb-girdle muscular dystrophy maps to chromosome 15 by linkage*. Comptes Rendus de l'Academie des Sciences (Paris) 1991; 312 series III:141-8.

[86] Speer MC, Yamaoka LH, Gilchrist JM, et al. *Localisation of an autosomal dominant form of limb-girdle muscular dystrophy to chromosome 5q*. Human genome mapping 1991; 11:abstract 26929.

[87] Romeo G, Roncuzzi L, Sangiorgi S, et al. Mapping of the Emery-Dreifuss gene through reconstruction of crossover points in two Italian pedigrees. *Hum Genet* 1988; 80:59-62.

[88] Specht LA, Beggs AH, Korf B, et al. Prediction of dystrophin phenotype by DNA analysis in Duchenne/Becker muscular dystrophy. *Ped Neurol* 1992; 8:432-6.

[89] Ahn AH, Kunkel LM. The structural and functional diversity of dystrophin. *Nature* Genetics 1993; 3:283-91.

[90] Koenig M, Monaco AP, Kunkel LM. The complete sequence of dystophin predicts a rod-shaped cytoskeletal protein. *Cell* 1988; 53:219-26.

[91] Bushby KMD. Recent advances in understanding muscular dystrophy. *Arch Dis Childhood* 1992; 67:1310-2.

[92] Mongini T, Palmucci L, Doriguzzi C, et al. Absence of dystrophin in two patients with Becker type Xp21 muscular dystrophy. *Neurosci Letters* 1992; 147:37-40.

[93] Hoffman EP, Fischbeck KH, Brown RH, et al. Characterization of dystrophin in muscle biopsy specimens from patients with Duchenne's or Becker's muscular dystrophy. *New Engl J Med* 1988; 318:1363-8.

[94] Hoffman EP. Myoblast transplantation: What's going on? *Cell Transplantation* 1993; 2:49-57.

[95] Chen M, Li HJ, Fang Q, et al. Dystrophin cytochemistry in mdx mouse muscles injected with labeled normal myoblasts. *Cell Transplantation* 1992; 1:17–22.

[96] Partridge TA, Morgan JE, Coulton GR, et al. Conversion of mdx myofibers from dystrophin-negative to -positive by injection of normal myoblasts. *Nature* 1989; 337:176–9.

[97] Karpati G, Pouliot Y, Zubrzycka-Gaarn, et al. Dystrophin is expressed in mdx skeletal muscle fibers after normal myoblast implantation. *Am J Pathol* 1989; 135:27-32.

[98] Law PK, Bertorini TE, Goodwin TG, et al. Dystrophin production induced by myoblast transfer therapy in Duchenne muscular dystrophy. *Lancet* 1990; 336:114–5.

[99] Law PK, Goodwin TG, Fang Q, et al. Myoblast transfer therapy for Duchenne muscular dystrophy. *Acta Paediatr Jpn* 1991; 33:206–15.

[100] Law PK, Goodwin TG, Fang Q, et al. Pioneering development of myoblast transfer therapy. In: Angelini C et al. (eds). *Muscular Dystrophy Research*. New York: Elsevier Science Publishers, 1991:109–16.

[101] Law PK, Goodwin TG, Fang Q, et al. Long-term improvement in muscle function, structure and biochemistry following myoblast transfer in DMD. *Acta Cardiomiologica* 1991; 1:281–301.

[102] Gussoni E, Pavlath GK, Lanctot AM, et al. Normal dystrophin transcripts detected in Duchenne muscular dystrophy patients after myoblast transplantation. *Nature* 1992; 356:435–8.

[103] Tremblay JP, Malouin F, Roy R, et al. Results of a triple blind clinical study of myoblast transplantations without immunosuppressive treatment in

young boys with Duchenne muscular dystrophy. *Cell Transplantation* 1993; 2:99–112.

[104] Huard J, Bourchard JP, Roy R, et al. Myoblast transplantation produced dystrophin-positive muscle fibers in a 16-year-old patient with Duchenne muscular dystrophy. *Clin Sci* 1991; 81: 287–8.

[105] Huard J, Bouchard JP, Roy R, et al. Human myoblast transplantation: preliminary results of 4 cases. *Muscle Nerve.* 1992; 15:550-60.

[106] Acsadi G, Dickson G, Love DR, et al. Human dystrophin expression in mdx mice after intramuscular injection of DNA constructs. *Nature* 1991; 352:815–8.

[107] Wolff JA, Malone RW, Williams P, et al. Direct gene transfer into mouse muscle in vivo. *Science* 1991; 247:1465–8.

[108] Lee CC, Pons F, Jones PG, et al. Mdx transgenic mouse – restoration of recombinant dystrophin to the dystrophic muscle. *Human Gene Therapy* 1993; 4:273-81.

[109] Dunckley MG, Wells DJ, Walsh FS, et al. Direct retroviral-mediated transfer of a dystrophin minigene into mdx mouse muscle in vivo. *Human Molecular Genetics* 1993; 2:717-23.

[110] Ragot T, Vincent N, Chafey P. Efficient adenovirus-mediated transfer of a human minidystrophin gene to skeletal muscle of mdx mice. *Nature* 1993; 361:647-50.

[111] Cooper BJ. The xmd dog: molecular and phenotypic characteristics. In: Kakulas BA, Howell JM, Roses AD (eds). *Duchenne Muscular Dystrophy. Animal Models and Genetic manipulations.* New York: Raven Press, 1992:109-11.

[112] Hyde SC, Gill DR, Higgins CF, et al. Correction of the ion transport defect in cystic fibrosis transgenic mice by gene therapy. *Nature* 1993; 362:250-5.

[113] Cournoyer D, Caskey CT. Gene therapy of the immune system. *Annu Rev. Immunol.* 1993; 11:297-329.

[114] Jiao S, Williams P, Berg RK, et al. Direct gene transfer into nonhuman primate myofibers in vivo. *Human Gene Therapy* 1992; 3:21-33.

[115] Wolff JA, Dority ME, Jiao S, et al. Expression of naked plasmids by cultured myotubes and entry of plasmids into t tubules and caveolae of mammalian skeletal muscle. *J Cell* Sci 1992; 103:1249-59.

[116] Xu H, Miller J, Liang BT. High-efficiency gene transfer into cardiac myocytes in vivo. *Trends Cardiovasc Med* 1991; 1:271-6.

[117] Leinwand LA, Leiden JM. Gene transfer into cardiac myocytes in vivo. *Trends Cardiovasc Med* 1991; 1:271-6.

[118] Caskey CT, Rossiter BJF. Molecular medicine. 9th Ernst Klenk Lecture. *Biol Chem Hoppe-Seyler* 1992; 373:159-70.

[119] Smith BF, Hoffman RK, Giger URS, Wolfe JH. Genes transferred by retroviral vectors into normal and mutant myobalasts in primary cultures are expressed in myotubes. *Mol Cell Bio* 1990; 10:3268-71.

[120] Dhawan J, Pan LC, Pavlath GK, et al. Systemic delivery of human growth hormone by injection of genetically engineered myoblasts. *Science* 1991; 254:1509-12.

[121] Barr E, Leiden JM. Systemic delivery of recombinant proteins by genetically modified myoblasts. *Science* 1991; 254:1507-9.

[122] Culver KW, Osborne WR, Miller AD, et al. Correction of ADA deficiency in human T lymphocytes using retroviral-mediated gene transfer. *Transplant Proc* 1991; 23: 170-1.

[123] Dickson G, Love DR, Davies KE, et al. Human dystrophin gene transfer: production and expression of a functional recombinant DNA-based gene. *Hum Genet* 1991; 88:53-8.

[124] Law PK. A consideration of the theoretical strategies which may minimize, ameliorate or correct the defect in DMD. In: Kakulas BA, Masaglia FL (eds). *Pathogenesis and Therapy of Duchenne and Becker Muscular Dystrophy*. New York: Raven Press, 1991:190.

[125] Acsadi G, Jani A, Massie B, et al. A differential efficiency of adenovirus-mediated in vivo gene transfer into skeletal muscle cells of different maturity. *Hum Mol Gen* 1994; 3:579-84.

[126] Neumeyer AM, DiGregorio DM, Brown RH Jr. Arterial delivery of myoblasts to skeletal muscle. *Neurology* 1992; 42:2258-62.

[127] Watson JD, Gilman M, Witkowski J, et al (eds). *Recombinant DNA*. New York: WH Freeman and Co., 1992:576.

[128] Lee CC, Pearlman JA, Chamberlain JS, et al. Expression of recombinant dystrophin and its localization to the cell membrane. *Nature* 1991; 349:334-6.

[129] Campbell KP, Kahl SD. Association of dystrophin and an integral membrane glycoprotein. *Nature* 1989; 338:259-62.

[130] Ervasti JM, Ohlendieck K, Kahl SD, et al. Deficiency of a glycoprotein component of the dystrophin complex in dystrophic muscle. *Nature* 1990; 345:315-9.

[131] Ervasti JM, Campbell KP. Membrane organization of the dystrophin-glycoprotein complex. *Cell* 1991; 66:1121-31.

[132] Ibraghimov-Beskrovnaya O, Ervasti JM, Leveille CJ, et al. Primary structure of dystrophin-associated glycoproteins linking dystropin to the extracellular matrix. *Nature* 1992; 355:696-702.

[133] Ohlendieck K, Matsumura K, Ionasescu VV, et al. Duchenne muscular dystrophy: deficiency of dystrophin-associated proteins in the sarcolemma. *Neurology* 1993; 43:795-800.

[134] Matsumura K, Nonaka I, Campbell K. Abnormal expression of dystrophin-associated proteins in Fukuyama-type congenital muscular dystrophy. *Lancet* 1993; 341:521-2.

[135] Matsumura K, Ervasti JM, Ohlendieck K, et al. Association of dystrophin-related protein with dystrophin-associated proteins in mdx mouse muscle. *Nature* 1992; 360:588-91.

[136] Roberds SL, Ervasti JM, Anderson RD, et al. Disruption of the dystrophin-glycoprotein complex in the cardiomyopathic hamster. *J Biol Chem* 1993; 268:11496-9.

[137] Hasty P, Bradley A, Morris JH, et al. Muscle deficiency and neonatal death in mice with a targeted mutation in the myogenin gene. *Nature* 1993; 364:501-6.

[138] Nobeshima Y, Hanaoka K, Hayacaka M, et al. Myogenin gene disruption results in perinatal lethality because of severe muscle defect. *Nature* 1993; 364:532-5.

[139] Anderson WF. Human gene therapy. *Science* 1992; 256:808-13.

[140] Matsumura K, Tome FMS, Ionasescu V, et al. Deficiency of dystrophin-associated proteins in Duchenne muscular dystrophy patients lacking COOH-terminal domains of dystrophin. *J Clin Invest* 1993; 92:866-71.

[141] Law PK, TG Goodwin, Q Fang, et al. Feasibility, safety, and efficacy of myoblast transfer therapy on Duchenne muscular dystrophy boys. *Cell Transplant* 1992; 1:235–44.

[142] Gage F, Christen Y (eds). *Gene transfer and therapy in the nervous system.* New York: Springer-Verlag; 1992.

[143] Kakulas BA, Mastaglia FL, eds. *Pathogenesis and Therapy of Duchenne and Becker Muscular Dystrophy.* New York: Raven Press, 1990: 1-273.

[144] Griggs RC, Karpati G, eds. *Myoblast Transfer Therapy. Adv Exp Med Biol.* New York: Plenum Press, 1990; 280:1-316.

[145] Law PK, Goodwin TG, Wang MG. Normal myoblast injections provide genetic treatment for murine dystrophy. *Muscle Nerve* 1988; 11:525-33.

[146] Law PK, Goodwin TG, Li HJ. Histoincompatible myoblast injection improves muscle structure and function of dystrophic mice. *Transplant Proc* 1988; 20:1114-9.

[147] Law PK, Li JH, Goodwin TG, et al. Pathogenesis and treatment of hereditary muscular dystrophy. In: Kakulas, BA, Mastaglia FL, eds. *Pathogenesis and therapy of Duchenne and Becker muscular dystrophy.* New York: Raven Press, 1990: 101-18.

[148] Law PK, Goodwin TG, Li HJ, et al. Myoblast transfer improves muscle genetics/structure/function and normalizes the behavior and life-span of dystrophic mice. In: Griggs RC, Karpati G, eds. *Myoblast Transfer Therapy.* New York: Plenum Press, 1990: 75-87.

[149] Konigsberg IR. Clonal analysis of myogenesis. *Science* 1963; 140:1273-84.

[150] Bischoff R. Regeneration of single muscle fibers in vitro. *Anat Rec* 1975; 182:215-26.

[151] Hauschka SD, Linkhart TA, Clegg C, et al. Clonal studies of human and mouse muscle. In: Mauro A, ed. *Muscle Regeneration.* New York: Raven Press, 1979: 311-22.

[152] Lyon MF. Gene action in X-chromosomes of the mouse (M. musculus L*).* *Nature* 1961; 190:372-3.

[153] Peterson AC. Chimaera mouse study shows absence of disease in genetically dystrophic muscle. *Nature* 1974; 248:561-4.

[154] Peterson AC, Pena S. Relationship of genotype and in vitro contractility in mdg/mdg – +/+ "mosaic" myotubes. *Muscle Nerve* 1984; 7:194-203.

[155] McComas AJ, Sica REP, Campbell MJ. 'Sick' motoneurones. A unifying concept of muscle disease. *Lancet* 1971; 1:321-5.

[156] Sica REP, McComas AJ. The neural hypothesis of muscular dystrophy. A review of recent experimental evidence with particular reference to the Duchenne form. *Can J Neurol Sci* 1978; 5:189-97.

[157] Bradley WG, Jaros E. Involvement of peripheral and central nerves in murine dystrophy. *Ann NY Acad Sci* 1979; 317:132-42.

[158] Okada E, Mizukira V, Nakamura H. Dysmyelination in the sciatic nerves of dystrophic mice. *J Neurol Sci* 1976; 28:505-20.

[159] Meier H, Southard JL. Muscular dystrophy in the mouse caused by an allele at the dy locus. *Life Sci* 1970; 9:137-44.

[160] Bulfield G, Siller WG, Wight PAL, et al. X chromosome-linked muscular dystrophy (mdx) in the mouse. *Proc Natl Acad Sci USA* 1984; 81:1189-92.

[161] Dangain J, Vrbova G. Muscle development in mdx mutant mice. *Muscle Nerve* 1984; 7:700-4.

[162] Coulton GR, Morgan JE, Partridge TA, et al. The mdx mouse skeletal muscle myopathy: I, a histological, morphometric and biochemical investigation. *Neuropath Appl Neurobiol* 1988; 14:53-70.

[163] Coulton GR, Curtin NA, Morgan JE, et al. The mdx mouse skeletal muscle myopathy: II, contractile properties. *Neuropath Appl Neurobiol* 1988; 14:299-314.

[164] Cooper BJ, Winand NJ, Stedman H, et al. The homologue of the Duchenne locus is defective in X-linked muscular dystrophy of dogs. *Nature* 1988; 334:154-6.

[165] Kornegay JN, Tuler SM, Miller DM, et al. Muscular dystrophy in a litter of golden retriever dogs. *Muscle Nerve* 1988; 11:1056-64.

[166] Sugita H, Arahata K, Tsukahara T, et al. Immunohistochemistry of dystrophin in various neuromuscular diseases. In: Kakulas BA, Mastaglia FL, ed. *Pathogenesis and Therapy of Duchenne and Becker Muscular Dystrophy*. New York: Raven Press, 1990:33-44.

[167] Partridge TA, Sloper JC. A host contributions to the regeneration of muscle grafts. *J Neurol Sci* 1977; 33:425-35.

[168] Partridge TA, Grounds M, Sloper JC. Evidence of fusion between host and donor myoblasts in skeletal muscle grafts. *Nature* 1978; 273:306-8.

[169] Law PK, Yap JL. New muscle transplant method produces normal twitch tension in dystrophic muscle. *Muscle Nerve* 1979; 2:356-63.

[170] Jones PH. Implantation of cultured regenerate muscle cells into adult rat muscle. *Exp Neurol* 1979; 66:602-10.

[171] Law PK. Beneficial effects of transplanting normal limb-bud mesenchyme into dystrophic mouse muscle. *Muscle Nerve* 1982; 5:619-27.

[172] Ontell M. Muscular dystrophy and muscle regeneration. *Hum Path* 1986; 17:673-82.

[173] Watt DJ. Factors which affect the fusion of allogeneic muscle precursor cells in vivo. *Neuropath Appl Neurol* 1982; 8:135-47.

[174] Watt DJ, Lambert K, Morgan JE, et al. Incorporation of donor muscle precursor cells into an area of muscle regeneration in the host mouse. *J Neurol Sci*. 1982; 57:319-31.

[175] Watt DJ, Morgan JE, Partridge TA. Long-term survival of allografted muscle precursor cells following a limited period of treatment with cyclosporin A. *Clin Exp Immunol* 1984; 55:419-26.

[176] Morgan JE, Watt DJ, Sloper JC, et al. Partial correction of an inherited biochemical defect of skeletal muscle by grafts of normal muscle precursor cells. *J Neurol Sci*. 1988; 86:137-47.

[177] Morgan JE. Practical aspects of myoblast implantation: investigations on two inherited myopathies in animals. In: Griggs RC, Karpati G, eds. *Myoblast Transfer Therapy*. New York: Plenum Press, 1990:89-96.

[178] Kornegay JN, Prattis SM, Bogan DJ, et al. Results of myoblast transplantation in a canine model of muscle injury. In: Kakulas BA, Howell JMC, Roses AD, eds. Duchenne muscular dystrophy. *Animal models and genetic anipulation.* New York:Raven Press, 1992:203-12.

[179] Carter ND, Parr CW. Isoenzymes of phosphoglucose isomerase in mice. *Nature* 1967;216:511.

[180] Chapman VM, Whitten WK, Ruddle FH. Expression of aternal glucose phosphate isomerase-1 (Gpi-1) in preimplantation stages of mouse embryos. *Dev. Biol* 1971;26:153-8.

[181] Padua RA, Bulfield G, Peters J: Biochemical genetics of a new glucosephosphate isomerase allele (Gpi-1c) from wide mice. *Biochem Genet* 1978;16:127-43.

[182] Gearhart JD, Mintz B. Clonal origins of somites and their muscle derivations: evidence from allophenic mice. Dev Biol 1972; 29:27-37.

[183] Watt DJ, Morgan JE, Partridge TA. Use of mononuclear precursor cells to insert allogeneic genes into growing mouse muscles. *Muscle Nerve* 1984; 7:741-50.

[184] Frair PM, Peterson AC. The nuclear-cytoplasmic relationship in "mosaic" skeletal muscle fibers from mouse chimaeras. *Exp Cell Res* 1983; 145:167-78.

[185] Blau HM, Chiu CP, Pavlath G, et al. Muscle gene expression in heterokaryons. *Adv. Exp. Med. Biol.* 1985;182:231-47.

[186] Wang MG, Law PK. Activity levels and preparative electrophoresis of GPI-1BB and GPI-1CC in host and donor mouse solei. *Proc Intl. Union. Physiol. Sci.* 1986;16:14.

[187] Li HJ, Wang MG, Goodwin TG, et al. Purification of mouse muscle GPI-1BB and GPI-1CC for antibody production. *Soc Neurosci Abst* 1986; 12:1289.

[188] Li HJ, Chen M, Goodwin TG, et al. Immunocytochemical differentiation of glucosephosphate isomerase allotypes. *Soc Neurosci Abst* 1990;16:347.

[189] Fang Q, Chen M, Li HJ, et al. Vital marker for muscle nuclei in myoblast transfer *Can J Physiol Pharmacol* 1991;69:49-52.

[190] Friedlander M, Fischman DA. Immunological studies of the embryonic muscle cell surface. Antiserum to the pre-fusion myoblast. *J Cell Biol.*1979;81:193-214.

[191] Law PK, Goodwin TG, Fang Q, et al. Cell transplantation as an experimental treatment for Duchenne muscular dystrophy. *Cell Transplantation* 1993;2:485-505.

[192] Kahan BD, Bach JF, eds. Proceedings of the second international congress on cyclosporine. Therapeutic use in transplantation. *Transplant Proc* 1988; 20:1-1137.

[193] Starzl TE, Thomson AW, Todo SN, et al., eds. Proceedings of the first international congress on FK 506. *Transplant Proc* 1991; 23:2709-3380.

[194] Weller B, Massa R, Karpati G, et al. Glucocorticoids and imunosuppressants do not change the prevalence of necrosis and regeneration in mdx skeletal muscles. *Muscle Nerve* 1991; 14:771-4.

[195] Law, P.K., Li, H., Chen, M. et at. (1994). Myoblast injection methods regulates cell distribution and fusion. *Tranplant. Proc.* 26, 3417-3418.

[196] Law PK, Goodwin TG, Li HJ, et al. Plausible structural/functional/behavioral/ biochemical transformations following myoblast transfer therapy. In: Griggs R, Karpati G, eds. *Myoblast Transfer Therapy*. New York: Plenum Press, 1990:241-50.

[197] Hooper C. Duchenne therapy trials starting in U.S., Canada. *J NIH Res* 1990; 2:30.

[198] Law PK, Goodwin TG, Fang Q, et al. Myoblast transfer therapy for Duchenne muscular dystrophy. *Adv Clin Neurosci* 1992; 2:463-70.

[199] Roelofs RK, deArengo GS, Law PK, et al. Treatment of Duchenne muscular dystrophy and D,L-penicillamine: results of a double-blind trial. *Arch Neurol* 1979; 36:266-8.

[200] McComas AJ, Brandstater ME, Upton ARM, et al. Sick motor neurons and dystrophy: A reappraisal. In: Rowland LP, ed. *Pathogenesis of Human Muscular Dystrophies.* Amsterdam: Excerpta Medica, 1977:180-6.

[201] Thomson AW, ed. Sandimmune (Cyclosporin). *Mode of action and clinical application*. Boston: Kluwer, 1989:1-364.

[202] Kahan BD. Cyclosporine and transplantation. *Transplant Immunol Letter* 1988; 4:1-120.

[203] Hoffman EP, Watkins SC, Slayter HS, et al. Detection of a specific isoform of alpha-actinin with antisera directed against dystrophin. *J Cell Biol* 1989; 108:503-9.

[204] Bonilla E, Samitt CE, Miranda AF, et al. Duchenne muscular dystrophy: deficiency of dystrophin at the muscle cell surface. *Cell* 1988; 54: 447-52.

[205] Kolata G. Cell transplant found effective in muscle disease. Muscular dystrophy patient showed strength increase in first human test. *The New York Times, Sunday, June 3*, 1990; A1.

[206] Beardsley T. Profile:Gene doctor. W. French Anderson pioneers gene therapy. *Sci Am* 1990; 263:33-4.

[207] Anderson, WF: Editorial. September 14, 1990: The Beginning. *Hum Gene Ther* 1990; 1:371-2.

[208] Karpati G, Ajdukovic D, Arnold D, et al. Myoblast transfer in Duchenne muscular dystrophy. *Ann Neurol* 1993; 34:8-17.

[209] Karpati G. Myoblast transfer in Duchenne muscular dystrophy. A perspective. In: Angelini C, et al, eds. *Muscular Dystrophy Research*. New York: Elsevier Science Publishers, 1991:101-7.

[210] Miller RG, Pavlath G, Sharma K, et al. Myoblast implantation in Duchenne muscular dystrophy: the San Francisco study. *Neurology* 1992; 42:189-90.

[211] Caplan A, Carlson B, Faulkner J, et al: Skeletal muscle. In: Woo SLY, Buckwalter J, eds. *Injury and repair of the musculoskeletal soft tissues*. Park Ridge, IL: American Academy of Orthopaedic Surgeons, 1987:209-91.

[212] Aiameddine, H.S., Louboutin, J.P., Dehaupas, M. et al. (1994). Functional recovery induced by satellite cell grafts in irreversibly injured muscles. *Cell Transplantation 3*, 3-14.

[213] Albert, N., Tremblay, J.P. (1992). Evaluation of various gene transfection methods into human myoblast clones. *Transpl. Proc. 24*, 2784-2786.

[214] Alton, E.W.F.W. and Geddes D.M. (1994). Gene therapy for cystic fibrosis, a clinical perspective. *Gene Therapy 2*, 88-95.

[215] Anderson, W. F. (1995). Gene Therapy. *Scient. Amer. 273*, 96-98B.

[216] Appleyard, S. T., Dunn, M. 1., Dubowitz, V.et al. (1985). Increased expression of l-ILA ABC class I antigens by muscle fibres in Duchenne muscular dystrophy, inflammatory myopathy, and other neuromuscular disorders. *Lancet* 1, *361-363*.

[217] Brenner, M.K. (1995). Human somatic gene therapy progress and problems. *Int. Med. 237*, 22~-239.

[218] Brittberg, M., Lindahl, A., Nilsson, A. et al. (1994). Treatment of deep cartilage defects in the knee with autologous chondrocyte transplantation. *N. Engl. J. Med. 331*, 889-895.

[219] Carlson, B.M. (1983). *The regeneration and transplantation of skeletal muscle*. In, Seil, F. ed. Nerve, organ, and tissue regeneration, Research perspectives. Academic Press, New York. pp. 431-454.

[220] Chang, P. L. (ed). (1994*). Somatic Gene Therapy*. CRC Press. New York.

[221] Chen, 5.5., Chien, C.H., Yu, H.S. (1988). Syndrome of deltoid and/or gluteal fibrotic contracture; an injection myopathy. *Acta Neurol. Scand. 78*, 167-176.

[222] Chiu, R.C.J., Zibaitis, A., and Kao, R.L. (1995). Cellular cardiomyoplasty, myocardial regeneration with satellite cell implantation. *Ann. Thorac. Surg. 60*, 12-18.

[223] Coolican, S.A., Samuel, D.S., Ewton, D.Z. et al., (1997). The MTT ogenic and myogenic actions of insulin-like growth factors utilize distinct signaling pathways. 1. *Biol. Chem. 272*, 6653-6662.

[224] Cornetta, K., Morgan, R.A., Anderson, W.F. (1991). Safety issues related to retrovirus-mediated gene transfer in humans. *Hum. Gene Ther. 2*, 5-14.

[225] Coutelle, C., Caplen, N., Hart, S. et al. (1994). *Towards gene therapy for cystic fibrosis.* In Dodge, J.A., Brock, J.H., and Widdicombe, J.H., eds. Cystic Fibrosis Current Topics. John Wiley and Sons. New York. 2, 33-54.

[226] Crystal, R.G., McElvaney, N.G., Chu, C.S. et al. (1994). Administration of an adenovirus containing the human CFTR c DNA to the respiratory tract of individuals with cystric fibrosis. *Nature Genet. 8*, 42-5 1.

[227] Culver, K. W. (1996). *Gene Therapy, A Primer for Physicians.* Mary Ann Liebert, Inc.. Larchmont.

[228] Curiel, D. T., Pilewski, J. M., Albelda, S.M. (1996). Gene therapy approaches for inherited and acquired lung diseases. *Am. J. Respir. Cell Mol.* Bol. *14*, 1-18.

[229] Daar, A. S., Fuggle, S. Y., Fabre, 1. W. et al. (1984). The detailed distribution of l-ILA-A, B, C, antigens in normal human organs. *Transplantation 38*, 287-298.

[230] Dai, Y., Roman, M., Naviaus, R.K. et al. (1992). Gene therapy via primary myoblasts, long term expression of factor IX protein following transplantation in vivo. *Proc. Natl. Acad. Sci. USA 89*, 10892-10895.

[231] Davis, H.L., Whalen, R.G., Demeneix, B.A. (1993). Direct gene transfer into skelet al muscles in vivo, factors affecting efficiency of transfer and stability of experssion. *Hum. Gene Ther. 4*, 151- 159.

[232] Fang, Q., Chen, M., Li, H.J. etat. (1994). MHC-l antigens on cultured human myoblasts. *Transpl. Proc. 26*, 3467.

[233] Fex, S. and Jirmanova, I. (1969). Innervation by nerve implants of fast' and "slow" skelet al muscles of the rat. *Acta Physiol. Scand. 76*, 257-269.

[234] Guerette, B., Asselin, I., Vilquin, J.T, et al. (1995). Lymphocyte infiltration follwing allo. and xenomyoblast transplantation in mdx mice. *Muscle Nerve 18*, 39-51.

[235] Guerette, B., Skuk, D., Celestin, F. (1997). Prevention by Anti-LFA-1 of acute myoblast death following transplantation. *J. Immunol. 159*, 2522-2531.

[236] Hamamori, Y., Samal, B., Tian, J. etat. (1994). Persistent erythropoiesis by myoblast transfer of erythropoietin cDNA. *Hum. Gene Ther. 5*, 1349-1356.

[237] Heyck. H., Laudahn, G., Carsten, P.M. (1996).Enzymaktivitatsbestimmungen bei Dystrophia musculorum progressiva. In MTT teilung. *Klinisce Wochenschrift 44*, 695.

[238] Hillman, A. (1996) Gene Therapy: Socioeconomic and Ethical Issues: A Roundtable Discussion. Hum. *Gene Ther. 7*, 1139-1144.

[239] Hoeben, R.C. (1995). Gene therapy for the haemophilias current status. *The International Association o f Biological Standardization. 23*, 27-29.

[240] Hoffman, E.P., Brown, R.H., Kunkel, L.M. (1987). Dystrophin, the protein product of the Duchenne muscular dystrophy locus. *Cell 51*, 919-928.

[241] Huber, B. E., Lazo, J. S. (eds.) (1994). *Gene Therapy for Neoplastic Diseases*. The New York Academy of Sciences. New York.

[242] Jiao, S., Cheng, L., Wolff, l.A. et al. (1993). Particle mbardment-mediated gene transfer and expression in rat brain tissue. *Bio/Technology 11*, 497-502.

[243] Karlsson, S. (1991). Treatment of genetic defects in hematopoietic cell function by gene transfer. *Blood 78*, 248 1-2492.

[244] *Gene Therapy and Molecular Biology Vol 1*, 17

[245] Katagiri, T. Yamaguchi, A., Komaki, M. et al. (1994). Bone morphogenetic protien-2 converts the differentiation pathway of C2C12 myoblasts into the osteoblast lineage. *J. Cell Biol. 127*, 1755-1766.

[246] Kessler, D.A., Siegel, J.P., Noguchi, P.D. et al. (1993). Regulation of somatic cell-therapy and gene therapy by the Food and Drug Administration. *N. Engl. J. Med. 329*, 1169-1173.

[247] Kinoshita, I., Vilquin, J.T., Guerette, B. et al. (1994). Very efficient myoblast allotransplantation in mice under FK506 immunosuppression. *Muscle Nerve 17*, 1407- 1415.

[248] Knowles, M.R., Hohneker, K., Zhou, Z.Q. et al. (1995). A double blind vehicle-controlled study of adenoviral mediated gene transfer in the nasal epithelium of patients with cystic fibrosis. *N. Eng. J. Med. 333*, 823-831.

[249] Koh, G.Y., Soonpaa, M.H., Klug, M.G. et al. (1995). Stable fet al cardiomyocyte grafts in the hearts of dystrophic mice and dog. *J. Clin. Invest. 96*, 2034-2042.

[250] Langer, R, Vacanti, J.P. (1993). Tissue engineering. *Science 260*, 920-926.

[251] Lau, H.T., Yu, M., Fontana, A. et al. (1996). Prevention of islet allograft rejection with engineered myoblast expressing FasL in mice. *Science 273*, 109-112.

[252] Law, P.K. (1982). Beneficial effects of transplanting normal limb-bud mesenchyme into dystrophic mouse muscle. *Muscle Nerve 5*, 619-627.

[253] Law, P.K. (1994). *Myoblast Transfer: Gene Therapy for Muscular Dystrophy*. R.G. Landes Company, Austin, TX, p. 139-154.

[254] Law, P.K. and Atwood, H.L. (1972). Nonequivalence of surgical and natural denervation in dystrophic mouse muscle. *Exp. Neurol. 34*, 200-209.

[255] Law, P.K., Atwood, H.L., McComas, A.J. (1976). Functional denervation in the soleus muscle of dystrophic mice. *Exp. Neurol. 51*,434-443.

[256] Law, P.K., Bertorini, T.E., Goodwin, T.G. et al. (1990a). Dystrophin production induced by myoblast transfer therapy in Duchenne muscular dystrophy. *Lancet 336*, 114-115.

[257] Law, P.K., Goodwin, T.G., Fang, Q. et al. (1991b). Myoblast transfer therapy for Duchenne muscular dystrophy. *Acta Paediatr. Jpn. 33*, 206-215.

[258] Law, P.K., Goodwin, T.G. Fang, Q. et al. (1994a). Whole body myoblast transfer. *Transpl. Proc. 26*, 3381-3383.

[259] Law, P.K., Goodwin, T.G., Fang, Q. et al. (1995). Myoblast transfer, gene therapy for muscular dystrophy. *J. Cell Biochem*. p. 367.

[260] Law, P.K., Goodwin, T.G., Fang, Q. et al. (1996). Human gene therapy with myoblast transfer. *Mol. Biol. o f the Cell. 7*, 3639.

[261] Law, P.K., Goodwin, T.G., Fang, Q. et al. (1997a). Human gene therapy with myoblast transfer. *Transpl. Proc. 29*, 2234-2237.

[262] Law, P.K., Goodwin, T.G., Fang, Q., et al. (199 7b). First human myoblast transfer therapy continues to show dystrophin after 6 years. *Cell Transplantation 6*, 95-100.

[263] Law, P.K., Goodwin, T.G., Fang, Q. et al. (1997c). Myoblast transfer therapy (MTT) phase II clinical trials. *J Physiol. Biochem. 53*, 80.

[264] Law, P.K., Goodwin, T.G., Fang, Q. (1997d). Advances in clinical trials of myoblast transfer therapy (MTT*). J. Neurol. Sci. 150*, 5253.

[265] Law, P.K., Goodwin, T.G., Wang, M.G. (1988 b). Normal myoblast injections provide genetic treatment for murine dystrophy. *Muscle Nerve 11*, 525-533.

[266] In Kakulas, B.A., Mastaglia, F.L. eds. *Gene Therapy and Molecular Biology Vol 1*, 18

[267] Li, R. K., Jia, Z.Q., Weisel, R.D. et al. (1996). transplantation improves heart function. *Cardiomyocyte Ann Thorac. Surg. 62*, 654-661.

[268] Massimino, M.L., Rapizzi, E., Cantini, M. et al. (1997). ED2+ macrophages increase selectively proliferation in muscle cultures. *Biochem. Res. Comm. 235*,

[269] Mendell, J.R., Kissel, J.T., Amato, A.A. et. al. (1995). Myoblast transfer in the treatment of Duchenne muscular dystrophy. *N. Engl. 1. Med. 333*, 832-838.

[270] Miyanohara, A., Johnson, P.A., Elam, R.L. et al. (1992). Direct gene transfer to the liver with herpes simplex virus Type 1 vectors, transient production of physiologically relevant levels of circulating factor IX. *New Biol. 4*, 23 8-246.

[271] Morandi, L., Bemasconi, P., Gebbia, M. et al. (1995). Lack of mRNA and dystrophin epxression in DMD patients three months after myoblast transfer. *Neuromusc. Disord. 5*, 291-295.

[272] Morishita, R., Gibbons, G.H. Horiuchi, M. et al. (1995). A gene therapy strategy using a transcription factor decoy of the E2F binding site inhibits smooth muscle proliferation in vivo. *Proc. Natl. Acad. Sci. USA 92*, 5855-5859.

[273] Morsy, M.A., Caskey, C.T. (1997). Safe gene vectors made simpler. *Nature Biotech. 15*, 17.

[274] Murry, C.E., Wiseman, R.W., Schwartz, S.M. et al. (1996). Skeletal myoblast transplantation for repair of myocardial necrosis. *J. Clin. Invest. 98*, 2512-2523.

[275] Nerem, R.M., Sambanis, A. (1995). Tissue engineering from biology to biological substitutes. *Tissue Engineering 1*, 3-12.

[276] Partridge, T.A., Grounds, M., Sloper, J.C. (1978). Evidence of fusion between host and donor myoblasts in skelet al muscle grafts. *Nature 273*, 306-308.

[277] Puchalski, R.B., Fahl, W.E. (1992). Gene transfer by electroporation, lipofection, DEAE.dextran transfection compatibility with cell-sorting by flow cytometry. *Cytometry 13*, 23-30.

[278] Ray, I., Gage, F.H. (1992). Gene transfer in established and primary fibroblast cell lines, comparision of transfection methods and promoters. *Biotechniques 13*, 598-603.

[279] Robinson, S.W., Cho, P.W., Levitsky, H.I. et al. (1996). *Cell Transplantation 5*, 77-91.

[280] Rosenfeld, M.A. and Collins, F.S. (1996). Gene therapy for cystic fibrosis. *Chest 109*, 241-252.

[281] Sautter, C., Waldner, H., Neuhaus-Url, G. et al. (1991). Micro-targeting, high efficency gene transfer using a novel approach for the acceleration of micro-projectiles. *Rio/Technology 9*, 1080-1085.

[282] Schwartz, E.R. (1997). Tissue engineering focused AlP program. *Tissue Engineering 3*, 5-17.

[283] Smith, T.A.G., Mehaffey, M.G. Kavda, D.B. et al. (1993). Adenovirus mediated expression of therapeutic plasma levels of human factor IX in mice. *Nat. Genet. 5*, 397- 402.

[284] St. Louis, D., Verma, I.M. (1988). An alternative approach to somatic cell gene therapy. *Proc. Natl. Acad. Sc i. USA. 85*, 3150-3154.

[285] Stewart, M.J., Plautz, G.E., Del Buono, L. et al. (1992). Gene transfer in vivo with DNA-liposome complexes safety and acute toxicity in mice. *Hum. Gene Ther. 3*, 267-275.

[286] Sunada, Y., Bernier, S.M., Utani, A. et al. (1995). Identification of a novel mutant transcript of Iaminin a 2 chain gene responsible for muscular dystrophy and 2J dysmyelination in dy mice. *Hum. Mol. Genet. 4*, 1055-1061.

[287] Teboul, L., Gaillard, D., Staccini, (1995). Thiazolidinediones and fatty myogenic cells into adipose-like cells. *J. Biol. Chem. 270*, 28183-28187.

[288] Trubetskoy, V.S., Torchilin, V.P., Kennel, S.J. et al. (1992). Cationic liposomes enhance targeted delivery and expression of exogenous DNA mediated by N-terminal modified poly-L-lysine-antibody conjugate in mouse lung endothelial cells. Biochem. *Biophy. Acta. 1131*,311-313.

[289] Van Meter, C.H., Claycomb, W.C., Delcarpio, J.B. et al. (1995). Myoblast transplantation in the porcine model a potential technique for myocardial repair. 1. Thorac. *Cardiovasc. Surg. 110*, 1442-1448.

[290] Vilquin, J.T., Kinoshita, I, Roy, R. et al. (1995). Cyclosphosphamide immunosuppresion does not perM T T successful myoblast allotranplantation in mouse.Neuromus. *Disord. 5*, 511-517.

[291] Wolft~ l.A., Malone, R.W., Williams, P. et al. (1990). Direct gene transfer into mouse muscle in vivo. *Science 247*, 1465-1468.

[292] Wolff, l.A., Williams, P., Ascadi, G. et al. (1991). Conditions affecting direct gene transfer into rodent muscle in vivo. *Biotechniques 11*, 474-485.

[293] Yao, S.N., SM T T h, K.J., Kurachi, K. (1994). Primary myoblast-mediated gene transfer, persistent expression of human factor IX in mice. *Gene Ther. 1*, 99-107.

[294] Ishikawa F et al. "Nuclear proteins that bind the pre-mRNA 3' splice site sequence r(UUAG/G) and the human telomeric DNA sequence d(TTAGGG)In", *Molecular Cell Biology, 13*: 4301-4310,1993.

[295] Atkins B Z et al. Myogenic cell transplantation improves in vivo regional performance in infarcted rabbit myocardium. *J. Heart Lung Transplant 18*: 1173 – 1180,1999.

[296] Murry C E et al. Muscle cell grafting for the treatment and prevention of heart failure. *J. Card. Fail. 8*: S532 – S541,2002.

[297] Tang G H, et al. Cell transplantation to improve ventricular function in the failing heart. *Eur. J. Cardiothoracic Surg. 23*: 907 – 916,2003.

[298] Taylor D A, et al. Regenerating functional myocardium: Improved performance after skeletal myoblast transplantation. *Nat. Med. 4*: 929 – 933, 1998.

[299] Hamano K, et al. Therapeutic angiogenesis induced by local autologous bone marrow cell implantation. *Ann. Thoracic Surg. 73*: 1210 – 1215, 2002.

[300] Chedrawy E G et al. Incorporation and integration of implanted myogenic and stem cells into native myocardial fibers: Anatomic basis for functional improvements. *J. Thorac Cardiovasc Surg 124*: 584 – 590, 2002.

[301] Tomita S et al. Improved heart function with myogenesis and angiogenesis after autologous porcine bone marrow stromal cell transplantation. *J. Thorac Cardiovasc Surg 123*: 1132 – 1140, 2002.

[302] Chekanov V, and Kipshidze, N. Angiogenesis by means of endothelial cell transplantation. *J. Thorac Cardiovasc Surg 125*: 441 – 442,2003.

[303] Hamano K et al. Local implantation of autologous bone marrow cells for therapeutic angiogenesis in patients with ischemic heart disease. *Jpn. Circ. J. 65*:845 – 847, 2001.

[304] Sakai T et al. The use of ex vivo gene transfer based on muscle-derived stem cells for cardiovascular medicine. *Trends Cardiovasc Med 12*: 115 – 120, 2002.

[305] Suzuki K et al. Cell transplantation for the treatment of acute myocardial infarction using vascular endothelial growth factor-expressing skeletal myoblasts. *Circulation 104*: I207 – I212,2001.

[306] Tse H F et al. Angiogenesis in ischemic myocardium by intra-myocardial autologous bone marrow mononuclear cell implantation. *Lancet 361*: 47 – 49,2003.

[307] Yau T M et al. Enhanced myocardial angiogenesis by gene transfer with transplanted cells. *Circulation 104*: I218 – I222,2001.

[308] Atkins B Z. Results of cellular therapy for ischemic myocardial dysfunction. *Minerva Cardioangiol. 50*: 333 – 341,2002.

[309] Reinlib, L., and Field, L. Cell transplantation as future therapy for cardiovascular disease? A Workshop of the National Heart, Lung and Blood Institute. *Circulation 101*:e182 – e187,2002.

[310] Al Attar N et al. Long-term (1 year) functional and histological results of autologous skeletal muscle cells transplantation in rat. *Cardiovasc Res. 58*: 142 – 148,2003.

[311] Henningson C T et al. Embryonic and adult stem cell therapy. *Allergy Clin. Immunol. 111(2 Suppl.)*: S745 – S753,2003.

[312] Hutcheson K A et al. Comparison of benefits on myocardial performance of cellular cardiomyoplasty with skeletal myoblasts and fibroblasts. *Cell Transplant 9*: 359 – 368,2000.

[313] Kim W G et al. Autologous cardiomyocyte transplantation in an ovine myocardial infarction model. *Int. J. Artif. Org. 25*: 61 – 66,2002.

[314] Scorsin M et al. Comparison of the effects of fetal cardiomyocyte and skeletal myoblast transplantation on post infarction left ventricular function. *J. Thorac Cardiovasc.Surg 119*: 1169 – 1175,2000.

[315] Yoo K J et al. Autologous smooth muscle cell transplantation improved heart function in dilated cardiomyopathy. *Ann. Thorac Surg. 70*: 859 – 865, 2000.

[316] Yoo K J et al. Smooth muscle cells transplantation is better than heart cells transplantation for improvement of heart function in dilated cardiomyopathy. *Yonsei Med. J. 43*: 296 – 303,2002.

[317] Reffelmann T et al. Transplantation of neonatal cardiomyocytes after permanent coronary artery occlusion increases regional blood flow of infarcted myocardium. *J Mol Cell Cardiol 35*: 607 – 613,2003.

[318] Rubart M P et al. Physiological coupling of donor and host cardiomyocytes after cellular transplantation. *Circ. Res. 92*: 1217 – 1224,2003.

[319] Hagege A A et al. Viability and differentiation of autologous skeletal myoblast grafts in ischemic cardiomyopathy. *Lancet 361*: 491 – 492,2003.

[320] Pagani F D et al. Autologous skeletal myoblasts transplanted to ischemiadamaged myocardium in humans: Histological analysis of cell survival and differentiation. *J. Am. Coll. Cardiol. 41*: 879 – 888,2003.

[321] Ghostine S et al. Long-term efficacy of myoblast transplantation on regional structure and function after myocardial infarction. *Circulation 106*: I131 – I136,2002.

[322] Jain, M., et al. (2001). Cell therapy attenuates deleterious ventricular remodeling and improves cardiac performance after myocardial infarction. *Circulation 103*:1920 – 1927.

[323] Rajnoch, C., Chachques, J. C., Berrebi, A., Bruneval, P., Benoit, M. O., and Carpentier,A. (2001). Cellular therapy reverses myocardial dysfunction. *J. Thoracic Cardiovasc. Surg. 121*: 871 – 878.

[324] Reinecke, H., Poppa, V., and Murry, C. E. (2002). Skeletal muscle stem cells do not trans-differentiate into cardiomyocytes after cardiac grafting. *J. Mol. Cell. Cardiol. 34*:241 – 249.

[325] Leobon, B., Garcin, I., Menasche, P., Vilquin, J. -T., Audiant, E., and Charpak, S. (2002).Myoblasts transplanted into rat infarcted myocardium

are functionally isolated from their host. *Proc. Natl. Acad. Sci. USA 100*: 7808 – 7811.

[326] P K Law, et al., "Myoblast transfer as a platform technology of gene therapy", Gene Therapy and Molecular Biology, 1: 345-363, 1998.

[327] P K Law, "Myoblast transfer as a platform technology of gene therapy", Regulatory Affairs Focus, (Technology), 4: 25-27, 1999.

[328] P K Law, "Nuclear transfer and human genome therapy", Business Briefing – Future Drug Discovery (Genomics), pp. 38-42, Dec. 2001.

[329] Chilian WM (2003) Editorial Comment on Arteriogenesis – is this terminology necessary? *Basic Res Cardiol 98*: 6–7

[330] Ferrara N (2001) Role of vascular endothelial growth factor in regulation of physiological angiogenesis. *Am J Physiol Cell Physiol 280*: C1358–C1366

[331] Freedman SB, Isner JM (2002) Therapeutic angiogenesis for coronary artery disease. *Ann Int Med 136*: 54–71

[332] Haider Kh H et al. (2002) Human myoblast carrying hVEGF165 as cellular assist device for myocardial therapeutics. *Circulation 106*: II-148

[333] Hockel M, Schlenger K, Doctrow S, Kissel T, Vaupel P (1993) Therapeutic angiogenesis. *Arch Surgery 128*: 423–429

[334] Hojo Y et al. (2000) Expression of vascular endothelial growth factor in patients with acute myocardial infarction. *J Am Coll Cardiol 35*: 968–973

[335] Iwakura A et al. (2000) Myocardial ischemia enhances the expression of acidic fibroblast growth factor in human pericardial fluid. *Heart and Vessels 15*:112–116

[336] Kalka C et al. (2000) VEGF gene transfer mobilizes endothelial progenitor cells in patients with inoperable coronary disease. *Ann Thorac Surg 70*: 829–834

[337] Shibuya M, Ito N, Claesson-Welsh L (1999) Structure and function of vascular endothelial growth factor receptor-1 and-2. Curr Top and functional restoration. *Eur Heart J 24*: 404–411

[338] Zachary I, Mathur A, Yla-Herttuala S, Martin J (2000) Vascular protection: a novel non-angiogenic cardiovascular role for vascular endothelial growth factor. *Arterioscler Thromb Vasc Biol 20*:1512–1520

[339] Venter, J C et al., "The sequence of the human genome", *Science* 2001, 291: 1,304-351.

[340] *"Nuclear Structure and Gene Expression"*, ed. by R C Bird, G S Stein, J B Lian, J L Stein, Academic Press 1997, pp. 1-296.

[341] Law, P K et al., "World's first human myoblast transfer into the heart", *Frontiers in Physiology, p. A85, 2000.

[342] Law P K, "Compositions for and methods of treating muscle degeneration and weakness", *U.S. Patent No. 5,130,141, issued July 14*, 1992.

[343] Law P K, "Myoblast therapy for mammalian diseases", *Singapore Patent No. 34490 (WO 96/18303), issued August 22*, 2000.

[344] Menasche P, et al., "Early results of autologous skeletal myoblast transplantation in patients with severe ischemic heart failure", *Circulation, 104*: II-598, 2001.

[345] Law P K, "Automated Cell Processor", *U.S. Patent No. 6,261,832, issued July 17*, 2001.

[346] Law P K, "Instrument for Cell Culture", *Singapore Patent No. 74036, issued December 14*, 2001.

[347] Barnes J D,Stamatiou D, Liew C C, "Construction of a human cardiovascular cDNA microarray: portrait of the failing heart", *Biochem Biophy Res Comm, 280*: 964-969, 2001.

[348] Law P K, et al., *"Mechanisms of myoblast transfer in treating heart failure"*, in Kimchi A ed. Advances in Heart Failure. New York: Medimont. 2002: 43-48.

[349] Law P K, "The regenerative heart", Business Briefing: PharmaTech 2002, pp. 65-70, Apr. 2002.

[350] Law P K, "Concomitant angiogenesis/myogenesis in the regenerative heart", Business Briefing: Future Drug Discovery, pp. 64-67, October 2002.

[351] Law, P K, et al., *" Myoblast genome therapy and the regenerative heart"*, in : Kipshidze N N and Serruys P W ed. Handbook of Cardiovascular Cell Transplantation. Martin Dunitz,UK. (2004) pp.241-258.

[352] Law, P K, et al., Human VEGF165-myoblasts produce concomitant angiogenesis/ myogenesis in the regenerative heart. *Mol Cell Biochem 263*: 173-178. 2004.

[353] Husnain Kh. Haider,et al., Myoblast Transplantation for Cardiac Repair: A Clinical Perspective. Mol Ther 9:14, 2004.

[354] Ye, L.,et al.,Therapeutic angiogenesis *Basic Res Cardiol 99*: 121 – 132, 2004.

[355] Niagara, M I, et al. Autologous skeletal myoblasts transduced with a new adenoviral bicistronic vector for treatment of hind limb ischemia. *J Vas Surg. 40*:775-785,2004.

[356] Arsic N, Zentilin L, Zacchigna S, Santoro D, Stanta G, Salvi A, et al. Induction of functional neovascularization by combined VEGF and angiopoietin-1 gene transfer using AAV vectors. *Mol Ther* 2003;7:450-9.

[357] Rando TA, Blau HM. Primary mouse myoblast purification, characterization, and transplantation for cell-mediated gene therapy. *J Cell Biol* 1994;125:1275- 87.

[358] Smythe GM, Grounds MD. Exposure to tissue culture conditions can adversely affect myoblast behaviors in vivo in whole muscle grafts: implications for myoblast transfer therapy. *Cell Transplant* 2000;9:379-93.

[359] Thurston G, Rudge JS, Ioffe E, Zhou H, Ross L, Croll SD, et al. Angiopoietin-1 protects the adult vasculature against plasma leakage. *Nat Med* 2000;6:460-3.

[360] Law P K et al. The world's first myoblast study of Type II diabetic patients. Bussiness Briefing : North American Pharmacotherapy 2004 - Issue 2,pp.

[361] Law PK. Myoblast transfer : gene therapy for muscular dystrophy. Austin: R G Landes 1994, 1-164.

[362] Yaffe D, Shainberg A, Dym H. Studies on the prefusion stage during formation of multinucleated muscle fibers in vitro. In: Banker BQ, Przybylski RJ, Van Der Meulen JP, et al., eds. *Research in muscle development and the muscle spindle*. Amsterdam: Excerpta Medica 1972: 110-21.

[363] Young HE, Carrino DA, Caplan AI. Histochemical analysis of newly synthesized and accumulated sulfated glycosaminoglycans during musculogenesis in the embryonic chick leg. *J Morph* 1989; 201:85-103.

[364] Vandenburgh HH, Karlisch P, Shansky J, et al. Insulin and IGF-I induce pronounced hypertropy of skeletal myofibers in tissue culture. *Amer J Physiol* 1991; 260:C475-84.

[365] Satoh A, Labrecque C, Tremblay JP. Myotubes can be formed within implanted adipose tissue. Transpl Proc 1992; 24:3017-19.

[366] Myerburg RJ, Kessler KM, Interian A, et al. Clinical and experimental pathophysiology of sudden cardiac death. In: Zipes DP, Jalife J, eds. *Cardiac electrophysiology. From cell to bedside.* Philadelphia: WB Saunders Company, 1990: 666-78.

[367] Iwata Y, Nakamura H, Mizuno Y, et al. Defective association of dystrophin with sarolemmal glycoproteins in the cardiomyopathic hamster heart. *FEBS Lett* 1993; 329:227-31.

[368] Iwata Y, Nakamura H, Fujiwara K, et al. Altered membrane-dystrophin association in the cardiomyopathic hamster heart muscle. *Biochem Biophys Res Com* 1993; 190:589-95.

[369] P Menasche, et al., "Myoblast transplantation for heart failure", *Lancet, 357*: 279-280, 2001.

INDEX

D

E

H

I